[FIND YOUR MOJO]

A BOOK BY LORRI ANN CODE
FOUNDER OF MAMA BOOTCAMP INC.

MAMA BOOTCAMP

CALIFORNIA | VIRGINIA

Published by CreateSpace, 2015
Text Copyright © Lorri Ann Code, 2015
Photographs Copyright © Various Authors, 2015

• • •

Design by a creative brain : Traecy Berryman
Photographs by Various Authors
Edited by Susan Reynolds
Printed in the United States of America by
CreateSpace

• • •

ISBN ISBN-13: 978-1519784117
ISBN-10: 1519784112

• • •

more information at mamabootcamp.com

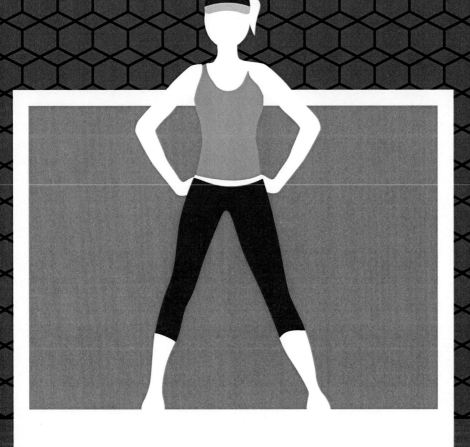

[FIND YOUR MOJO]

52 WEEKS TO TRANSFORMATION, INSPIRATION AND FITNESS

A BOOK BY LORRI ANN CODE
FOUNDER OF MAMA BOOTCAMP INC.

CONTENTS

FOREWORD

BY BETHANY CROUCH
ANCHOR, FOX40 NEWS

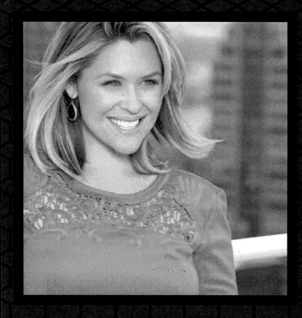

With tears streaming down her face, Lorri Ann Code stood in my living room. "I have to write this book. I have to write it so that other women know that there's a way out of the darkness." Lorri Ann Code; mother, wife, athlete, trainer, coach... agent of inspiration and proponent of the positive.

She is a force. She is relentless. She is inspiring.

Having known her since 2008 (after meeting at a live shot for the FOX40 morning show, in which I fell head over heels in love with her energy and enthusiasm), I'm thrilled Lorri Ann is choosing to share her incredible story in such a public way. However, putting that story on paper is to relive old traumas. Thus, the aforementioned tears in the living room.

Over years of long runs, bike rides, bootcamps, swims, hikes, retreats... Lorri Ann has shared her story and has blown me away. Despite core-quaking hurdles and heartbreaks, her courage, strength and resolve have only grown stronger. Through the hardship, Mama Bootcamp was born.

Lorri Ann is driven by a passion to help people push themselves to new limits, break old destructive cycles and emerge with new self-confidence and self-love. It's the story of Lorri Ann's personal journey, and it can be your journey, too, as you get to know her in the pages that follow.

In her own words, Lorri Ann says "this book gives you practical, simple, and sometimes magical tools to help build a life you love. It's a year-long guide to motivate and inspire you to transform your life physically, emotionally, and spiritually."

This is a book about making good choices and creating the best life you can, no matter what your story is up to this point.

— BETHANY CROUCH

INTRODUCTION

BY LORRI ANN CODE
FOUNDER OF MAMA BOOTCAMP

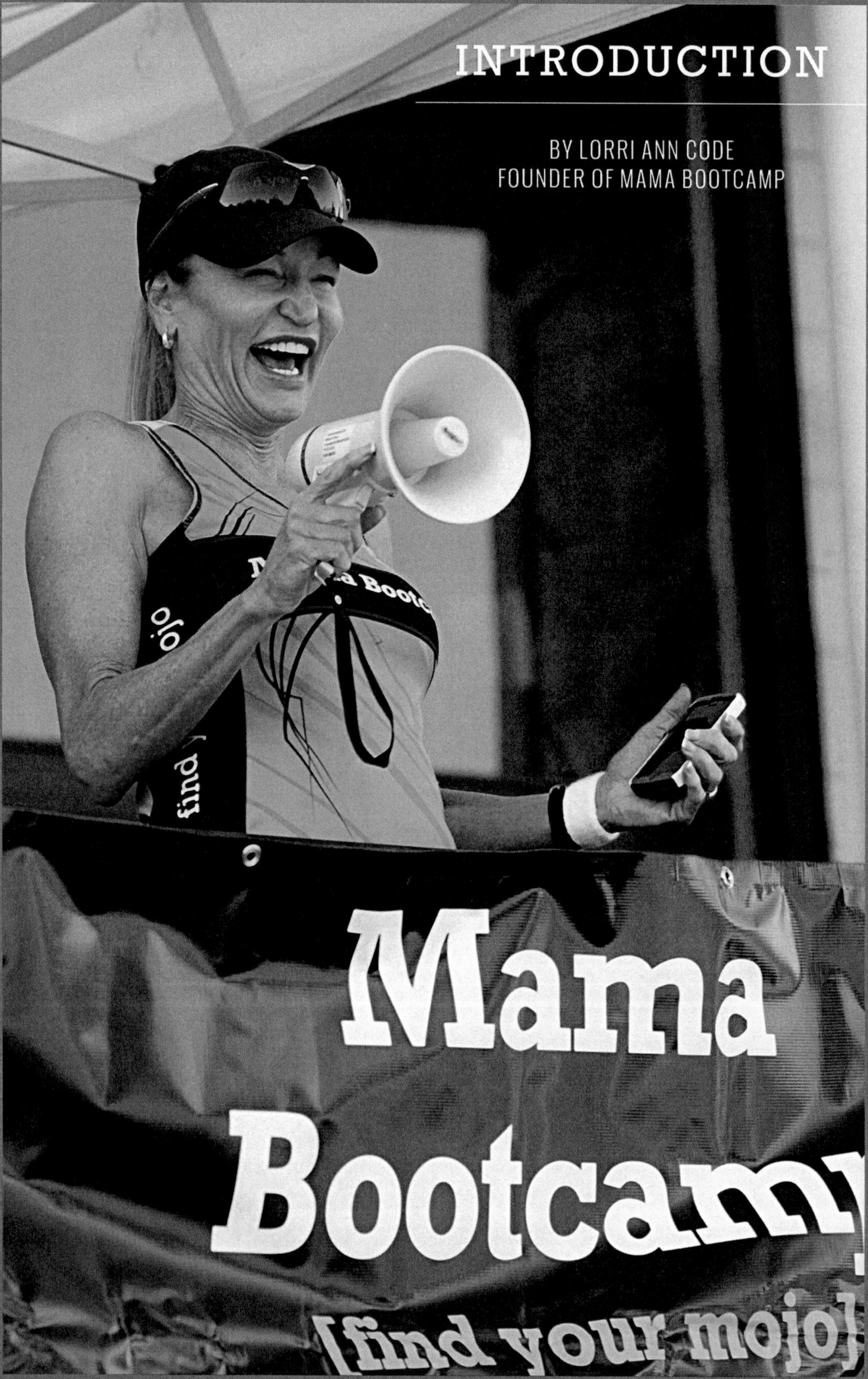

Y ou might be asking what is your "mojo" and why in the world would you ever want to find it? Great question and one that I will answer with a story.

One of my dear friends, Michelle, was in and out of the hospital a few years ago and not doing well. Doctors were unsure of what was going on and could not come up with a diagnosis for treatment. Hearing she was back in the hospital, I went to visit her in the afternoon. The blinds were drawn and the room was dark. I looked for Michelle thinking she was in her bed under the covers, realizing as my eyes adjusted to the dark, that she actually was in the corner of the room upright in a chair, in too much pain to move. I walked over to her and she looked up at me. Seeing my baseball cap with the words on it "find your mojo", she started crying and said "I want my mojo back" in a weak tiny voice that I barely recognized. I knew immediately what she meant.

She was sick and tired of being sick and tired. Lost with no answers. Her energy for life was gone. Michelle's situation was an extreme one, but how she felt and the words she said to me were ones I have heard often from my "Mamas". Mamas are the women I have the honor of coaching in Mama Bootcamp, a fitness business I created that addresses not just the body but the mind and spirit as well.

What Michelle was feeling and saying to me seemed like a common denominator with lots of women and my Mamas. Often stretched too thin, taking care of their jobs, homes, cats and dogs, children, husbands, boyfriends, or partners, and putting everyone and everything before their own needs... they had lost their way. Wondering how they got to this place of exhaustion and surrender, "Mamas" come to me to help them re-claim their lives and find their mojo. "Mojo" is an intangible magical energy that creates passion for your life. It is what gets you out of bed in the morning, excited to start your day, motivated and inspired to get moving!

When looking at the big picture, "finding your mojo" can seem like a daunting task and overwhelming. I want you focused, energized and inspired, but not overwhelmed! So where do you start? Being the leader and creator of mojo and motivation, I have broken it down into three color-coded pieces:

LIFE COACHING: TO MOTIVATE AND INSPIRE **[FUSHIA]**
FITNESS: TO GET THE BODY MOVING AND ENERGIZED **[BLUE]**
NUTRITION: FOCUSED ON CLEAN AND HEALTHY EATING IS BASED ON SIMPLICITY **[GREEN]**

Each month covers one of these areas with weekly challenges focusing on a story and an Action Plan. Keeping it simple is one of the major cornerstones of Mama Bootcamp and "finding your mojo". This year-long transformation is an adventure and a challenge. It will take follow through and commitment on your part, but what waits for you on the other side of the 52 weeks is a life that is worth living, a life you love.

Read through the book first making note of the challenges that hit home. You will be drawn to certain areas depending on where you are in your life, but there are some "back to basics": hydration, eating your veggies, getting enough sleep. It will be very difficult to find your mojo if you are dehydrated, malnourished, and exhausted!

This book is designed to jump in at any time... Even if you turn a small weekly challenge, such as hydration, into a lifestyle change, it will have huge impact on your life! Just keep moving through the challenges and stay committed and focused to your bigger goal: designing a life that you are happy to be living.

— LORRI ANN CODE

JANUARY

LIFE COACHING: CHOOSE WHERE YOU LIVE

[CHALLENGE 1]
A MANTRA TO MOVE THROUGH LIFE

[CHALLENGE 2]
CREATE A VISION BOARD

[CHALLENGE 3]
DEVELOP AN ATTITUDE OF GRATITUDE

[CHALLENGE 4]
MIRROR WORK

STARTING A NEW YEAR IS A REBIRTH OF SORTS FOR ME. IT IS A CHANCE TO CLEANSE, WITH A CLEAN SLATE TO RE-CREATE A WORLD I WANT TO LIVE IN. JANUARY WEEKLY CHALLENGES ARE FUN, EMPOWERING, CREATIVE, VISUAL, AND ARE LIFE CHANGING. I CHALLENGE YOU TO JUMP IN WITH BOTH FEET. HERE WE GO!

[CHALLENGE 1] MANTRA TO MOVE THROUGH LIFE

Every year, I pick a mantra, which is a phrase or word to represent the year and how I want to live it! I make business, personal, and life decisions around that word. Words in the past have been: fearless, believe, empowered, strength… and they definitely helped me be a better version of myself just by the power of the word.

One year my word was "faith" because I had lost all faith the previous year. I was totally on my knees after being betrayed by people who I thought were "family." The rug was ripped out from beneath me. I was honestly not sure I could get up again.

I felt broken with my soul deeply bruised. I needed to learn to trust myself.

How did I end up down a dark alley with people who wanted to destroy me? I chose them. It was completely and utterly baffling to me. I honestly just wanted to give up. If this was the world, then it was too painful for me and I wanted out.

I came home from a particularly rough day and told my husband I was going to ask my business partner to let me out of my partnership. I didn't know what I wanted to do (other than crawl in a dark hole and die.) Fortunately, my husband Les had faith in me when I did not. He said, "I know you. You will figure it out."

Simple but powerful words I leaned on until I could believe it myself. That next year was about rebuilding my faith. I looked for the red flags in every decision I made. I listened to my inner voice that would warn me, nudging about situations, business decisions, and people I allowed in my inner circle. I learned I could trust myself.

I challenged my Mamas to do the same and pick a word or phrase to live by. One of my coaches, Lori picked "committed." I love how she had chosen to use this word in her training for a triathlon. Running hill repeats one day, we were on our fifth hill and she shouted to me with a big smile on her face "I am committed" to finishing six hills today!" I loved hearing her enthusiasm, pride, and confidence proclaimed while pushing herself through to complete the hill! It was awesome! It is amazing what your one word can do.

ACTION PLAN NO. 1

Start thinking what happened this year. Where did you thrive and where did you nose dive? Are you proud of how you are living? Where would you like to see change?

Pick a word or phrase for the next year and what you want for yourself, your relationships, and your career. Pick your word or phrase carefully and intentionally. Decide to make decisions around that word. This is an easy and fun activity, but not so easy to move through a whole year living up to your "word" or "phrase":

FAITH	SERENITY	FEARLESS
BELIEVE	DETERMINED	STRENGTH
CALM	PEACE	COURAGE
JOY	PROSPERITY	LOVE
FOCUS	ABUNDANCE	FLOW

LIVING LIFE WITH PASSION OR PURPOSE.
LIVE, LAUGH, LOVE.
I CAN.
SHE THOUGHT SHE COULD SO SHE DID.
I AM EMPOWERED.

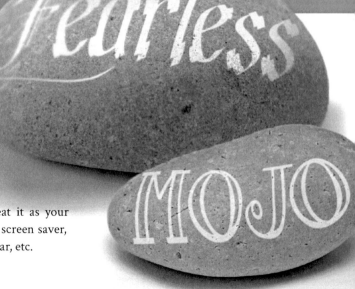

What do you do with this mantra? You design your life using it as your guiding light, directing you both personally and professionally. When you have a decision to make – ask if it is in alignment with your mantra for the year.

Put it in a place where you will repeat it as your mantra – on your phone, post-it notes, screen saver, 3x5 index cards, on your desktop calendar, etc.

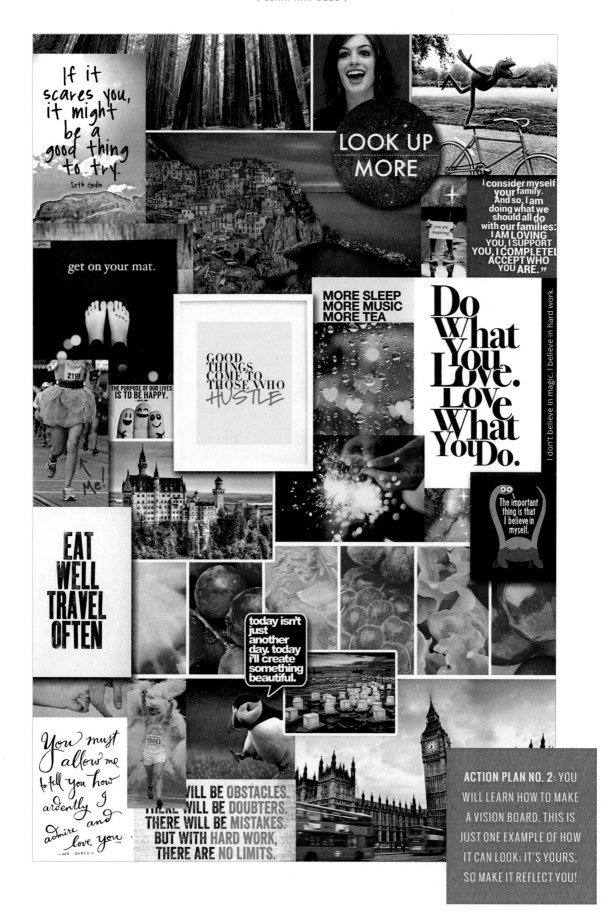

[CHALLENGE 2] CREATE A VISION BOARD

January is all about creation. For this challenge, you will be creating a life by designing a vision board or dream board. In my experience this is a huge tool for manifestation. We are only limited by what our brains can comprehend.

My vision boards have moved me for an abused single mother on welfare with three small children to an empowered independent, strong woman who owns her own successful corporation. It opened the window of my mind to the unlimited possibilities that exist and truly helped me to create a life I love and am passionate about.

ACTION PLAN NO. 2

SUPPLIES NEEDED:

POSTER BOARD	PICTURES FROM MAGAZINES OR WEBSITES THAT MOTIVATE/INSPIRE YOU	WORDS FROM MAGAZINES/ WEBSITES TO INSPIRE YOU
COLORED MARKERS/ COLORED PENCILS		
CONSTRUCTION PAPER	PICTURES OF FRIENDS/ FAMILY MEMBERS THAT INSPIRE YOU	PHOTOS OF YOU WHEN YOU FELT AND LOOKED YOUR BEST
GLUE, STICKERS, GLITTER		

Divide the board into areas you would like to grow, change, or manifest "more."

Allow yourself to dream BIG. This can be a very fun, creative, empowering dynamic process and hugely impactful.

Some areas to think about: ideal friendships, dream career, comforts of home, harmonic family, fitness goals (first 5K or triathlon), dream vacations, jewelry, write a check to you (how much do you want to make annually?).

This can be emotional, tangible or intangible. For example: What kind of car do you drive? Where do you want to live? How do you want to look? What would you like to do with your friends or family?

Find a quiet space and time to work on your board. Light candles, play music and let inspiration guide you.

Post your finished board somewhere where you can see it daily.

[CHALLENGE 3] DEVELOP AN ATTITUDE OF GRATITUDE

Whatever you focus on grows. What you "think about, comes about." Living in thankfulness creates a wondrous sense of joy and a synergistic "give and take" with life. This challenge is about being grateful.

What you give out definitely comes back to you. I won't lie, this is not the easiest of challenges. Some days are just HARD and the biggest thing to be thankful for may be that the day is over and you get to go to bed and "sleep it off." When I was having one of these bad days that turned into a bad week and then a bad month, I thought, "What is going on? What have I done to deserve this?!"

I forced myself to look at people who had much worse circumstances than I. People who couldn't go for a run to get rid of the stress or for whatever reason had no car to get to work. Not to relish in their misery, but to remind myself it could be worse.

Another way to be grateful is to help others who are down in their luck or to give back to others. You could pick up trash at a local park, work in a homeless shelter, volunteer at a hospital, or help a family in need. Doing something for others will move you through your temporary slump.

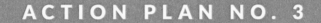

ACTION PLAN NO. 3

Purchase a journal and a nice pen. At the end of your day, name three things you are thankful for. Examples: I am thankful for my warm cozy bed. I am thankful for my supportive, loving husband. I am thankful for my coworkers. I am blessed with great neighbors. I have an amazing dog who is always happy to see me and offers unconditional love. I am thankful that I can go to bed and start over tomorrow.

At the end of the year, you will not only have a full year of gratitude, but all that wonderful energy comes back to you creating more good. This is very powerful. Look at how the year unfolds when you sprinkle your days with gratitude.

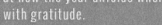
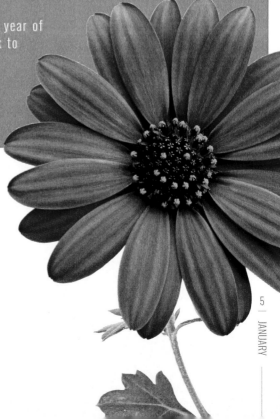

ACTION PLAN NO. 4

First, you will pick your affirmations. Choose statements that are in alignment with your mantra and your vision board. You are creating a life that you love and are passionate about. Dump ideas and thoughts that no longer serve you. Affirmations are short, powerful "I am" statements you say to yourself in the mirror looking into your own eyes. Make sure they are present tense as if it already is so.

Write your affirmations on 3 x 5 cards. Decorate if you like, but pull them out and read them to yourself until they are memorized. Examples:

I AM DESERVING OF A GREAT RELATIONSHIP.

I AM DESERVING OF A GOOD LIFE.

I AM HEALING AND BECOMING.

I AM LOVED.

I AM HEALTHY AND HAPPY.

I AM ABUNDANT.

I AM PROSPEROUS.

I AM FILLED WITH JOY.

I AM ABLE TO RELEASE MY PAIN.

I AM FLOWING THROUGH LIFE WITH PEACE, LOVE, AND HAPPINESS.

I AM STRONG AND CONFIDENT.

I AM EMPOWERED.

I AM ENERGIZED.

I AM PASSIONATE AND EXCITED ABOUT MY LIFE.

I AM EMOTIONAL, PHYSICALLY, AND MENTALLY STRONG.

Create the time or times in your day you will do your mirror work. Make it a priority. Early morning when you are just rolling out of bed is an especially effective time because you are open and receptive to hearing the words you say to yourself. They set the tone for the day and can be absorbed into your consciousness. In addition, things are less likely to get in your way and you will be consistent.

By doing your mirror work, you are dumping the junk (the mistruths told to you by people who had their own issues and problems) and reloading by choosing to be happy and healthy. The beauty of mirror work is that two things cannot occupy the same space at the same time. You are choosing to focus on creating what you want more of in your life!

Caution: Be aware of just "forgetting" to do your affirmations by oversleeping, avoiding your eyes, not making the time, or getting too busy. Choose to recommit to this very powerful process. It takes consistency on a daily basis for your subconscious to absorb the good soul food you are feeding it.

[CHALLENGE 4] MIRROR WORK

The combination of mirror work with affirmations can be a very powerful tool creating a huge meta-morphous in a short period of time. This depends on how much there is to "dump" and "reload." By this I mean, we all grow up with believing we are what our parents tell us we are. This can be great if you have healthy, loving parents or not so great if your parent are messed up themselves and live out their dysfunctions through you.

Two things cannot hold the same space at the same time, so dumping is a natural part of the process when you are reclaiming who you are. You came into this world perfect with natural inherent gifts that were meant to be shared. This is who you are. Growing up and being raised by parents who are critical and self-absorbed can cause you to feel unworthy and undeserving of life's abundance.

Bigger issues may manifest in all sorts of ways such as loneliness, sadness, low self-esteem, feeling unloved, and may cause low grade depression and worst. You are definitely not able to live your best life with bad programming that happened when you were your most vulnerable.

This work was the beginning for me of unloading a painful, chaotic, and confusing childhood. Having an absent dad who was gone all the time "working" and an alcoholic mother who could slice you and dice you in one fell swoop with her tongue was not a happy place.

On top of that, my mother wanted to be the center of attention and the one all her children "adored." In her misguided intent to do this, she would "pit" us against one another. My brother totally lost his way and gave up by falling head first into a battle with drugs which took him years to find his way out.

My sisters and I had no idea how to treat each other or how to have a loving relationship. We never saw it. The worst years were from age 10 to 16. I was a victim of molest, neglect, abandonment, betrayal and just felt like a foreigner in my own home. Our home was a scary, evil place. At 16 when I graduated from high school, I got the hell out and shared an apartment with a girlfriend. Looking back, I definitely was in survival mode and needed a safe place that I could claim as mine.

After suffering from a bout of depression, I knew I did not want to live with my childhood defining the rest of my life. One of the best tools I used to get back my life and reclaim my right to be happy was mirror work with affirmations.

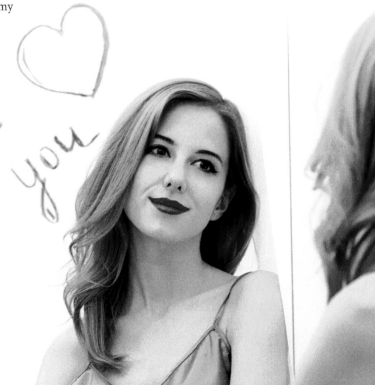

There is so much power in looking into your own eyes (the gateway to the soul) and affirming who you are or want to be. This maybe a challenge you do for a whole month, year, or ongoing depending on what you need or want to work on.

JANUARY IN REVIEW

FOR JANUARY
MY GOALS

FOR JANUARY
MY GRATITUDE LIST

FOR JANUARY
RELATIONSHIPS TO INVEST IN

FOR JANUARY
WHAT'S GOING WELL

FOR JANUARY
WHAT NEEDS TO CHANGE

MY DOODLE SQUARE

FEBRUARY

FITNESS:
BABY STEPS, BABY... BABY STEPS

WE STARTED THE YEAR WITH GETTING YOUR ATTITUDE ADJUSTED AND HEADING IN THE RIGHT DIRECTION TO BUILD YOUR FOUNDATION FOR YOUR BEST LIFE. AFTER ALL, THE FIRST STEP IS ADJUSTING WHAT GOES ON BETWEEN YOUR EARS. GETTING READY TO MAKE MAJOR LIFE CHANGES STARTS WITH A MIND SHIFT.

NOW LET'S GET MOVING!

[CHALLENGE 5] SMART GOALS

Goals are essential because without a plan to put into action, your goal becomes an unattainable wish. How many times have you said, "I wish I was in better shape" or "I wish I could run a 5K like my friends." Wishing will not make it so. You need to step into action! S.M.A.R.T. goals help by giving you an action plan that is achievable.

I had a client, Jane, who really wanted to get in great shape and to train for a half marathon. She printed our Mama Bootcamp half-marathon training plan and told her coach she was going to implement it into her schedule. A day went by and then a week and then months passed. The race came and went. Jane felt like a failure and beat herself up. She told me, "I don't know why I even try. I will never be a runner." She continued the negative self-talk and eventually stopped trying.

By not having a detailed plan that worked for her life and her schedule, she never implemented her training plan. It is so important to be specific on the steps you need to be successful. For Jane, she needed to commit to the days, times and places she was going to run and put them on her calendar. There was no detailed plan; no call to action.

Jane came back months later and decided to sit down with her coach and go over her calendar. We worked on time management and decided early morning runs were best. She asked her neighbor who had expressed an interested in also running a half marathon to train with her. They committed to each other to meet Mondays, Wednesdays, and Fridays at 5 am and run for thirty minutes. At the end of each run, Jane agreed to text me for accountability and progress reports. With her *big* goal and clear S.M.A.R.T. goals, Jane found the motivation and the accountability she needed to do the training and run in her first half-marathon! It was a huge confidence boost, too.

Remember, if your goal does not scare you a little, then it's not a big enough goal. So, think big or even bigger.

ACTION PLAN NO. 5

Today, right now, you are going to devise a plan that will have a start date. You will set S.M.A.R.T. goals. This is my version of S.M.A.R.T. Goals. They are:

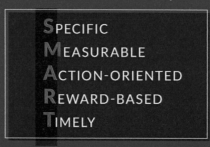

SPECIFIC
MEASURABLE
ACTION-ORIENTED
REWARD-BASED
TIMELY

USE THE GOAL SETTING WORKSHEET ON PAGES 14-15 TO CREATE CUSTOM S.M.A.R.T. GOALS.

STEP ONE: LONG-TERM GOALS

These are your big goals. What do you really want? What are your dreams? Refer back to your vision board.

STEP TWO: GOAL PHOTO

Find a picture of yourself when you looked and felt your best. This photo should be from when you were rocking your mojo, in the flow of life, and happy. Your goal photo should make you feel excited and energized. If you were super thin because you were going through a divorce or recovering from an illness, this would not be a good goal photo.

If you do not have a picture from a time in your life when you looked and felt great, then do a little research and find a picture from a magazine or website that inspires you. You will know it when you find it because it will hit your right between the eyes and heart. It will feel like: "I want THAT!"

STEP THREE: ANTICIPATED OBSTACLES

Problem solve conflicts and challenges ahead of time and have a plan to address those challenges. Are there donuts in the break room that call your name? Is it the vending machine at school? Does your girlfriend call you for "happy hour" weekly? Name them to know them. This way you are prepared to handle your challenges and move through them. Sometimes just recognizing the obstacle is enough to take power away from it.

STEP FOUR: MOTIVATION FACTOR

Why do you want to achieve your goal? Are you going on a big trip? Is it your class reunion? Is there a wedding in your future? Or are you training for life? All are great reasons to keep you moving toward this new life you are creating.

STEP FIVE: ACCOUNTABILITY

Get an accountability buddy so you have a person to report to. This can be a coach, personal trainer, a life coach,

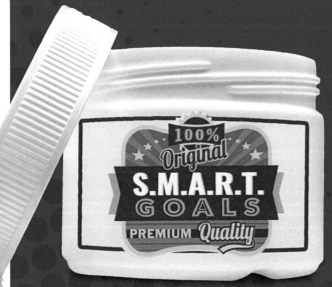

YOU CAN

a neighbor, a co-worker, a trusted friend, or a family member. Only share with those that will support your goals. Make sure to pick a buddy that is someone you trust not to "flake" on you. "Flaking" can be contagious and once your buddy "flakes" it sets up an unspoken agreement that it is okay to "not show up."

Caution: Do not share with someone who will sabotage you or who does not believe in you. There's no quicker way to destroy your dream than to throw your "pearls" before swine! (See Challenge No. 45).

STEP SIX: CONTINUED MOTIVATION

Keeping your eye on the prize: Make copies of your goal picture and post it around your house—on your bathroom mirror, your refrigerator, car visor, put it on post-it notes, make it your screen saver for your phone. The idea is to keep yourself focused. When you aim at nothing, that's what you get. When your sights are set on your goal, you can stay motivated and on track.

Be sure to reward yourself for a job well done along the way, not just at the completion of your big goal. Use small rewards for positive behavior changes to keep you going. It's the things you do daily that will lead you to your big goal. When you fall down (because you will...), get back up, dust yourself off, and refocus on your bigger goal.

STEP SEVEN: KNOWLEDGE OR SKILLS NEEDED

What do you need to know to get you to your goal? Do you need a 5K or half-marathon training plan? Do you need information on clean eating? Do you need to take classes at a local junior college to advance on your job? Do you need to download new apps for meditation? Seek out, research where you need help and get it.

STEP EIGHT: SMART GOALS AND REWARDS

Write three short-term goals related to achieving your big goal. Make sure your goals are specific, measurable, action oriented and timely. Complete your SMART goals with a deadline in mind. You need a call to action so you can get moving. You will also plan rewards for each goal.

The more detail in your goal, the more likely you are to attain the SMART goal. SMART goals are "action" oriented and long term is your vision. Your action plan is setting you up for success.

NOT S.M.A.R.T. GOALS	S.M.A.R.T. GOALS
I WILL DRINK MORE WATER. I WILL EAT MORE VEGGIES.	I WILL DRINK 40 OUNCES OF WATER BY NOON AND 40 OUNCES OF WATER BY 6 PM. I WILL HAVE A HOMEMADE SALAD FOR LUNCH AND PREPARE FIVE GRAB 'N GO'S BY 6 PM ON SUNDAY.

Reward yourself along the way for attaining your short term goals. Example: Your long term goal is to run a half marathon in June. Your first short term goal is to participate in a 5K race in March. Treat yourself to a pedicure after completion of the 5K race for a job well done.

Make your rewards fun and not food oriented. Other rewards include treating yourself to a massage, a new pair of running shoes, a movie with a friend, or sending the kids with dad and enjoying the solitude of a bubble bath with candles and music.

ACHIEVE YOUR BIG GOAL.

GOAL SETTING WORKSHEET

FIND A PHOTO OF YOURSELF WHERE YOU LOOK AND FEEL YOUR BEST,
OR FIND A PICTURE THAT INSPIRES YOU FROM A MAGAZINE, WEBSITE, ETC.
ATTACH IT TO THIS WORKSHEET.

NAME _____ DATE _____

LONG TERM GOAL _____
_____
_____
_____

PROJECTED
ACHIEVEMENT DATE

_____/_____/_____

ANTICIPATED OBSTACLES _____
_____
_____
_____

MOTIVATION FACTOR [WHY DO YOU WANT THIS?] _____
_____
_____

PERSON OR GROUP WHO WILL SUPPORT YOU AND HOLD YOU ACCOUNTABLE
_____

HOW WILL YOU CONTINUE TO MOTIVATE YOURSELF? _____
_____
_____

KNOWLEDGE OR SKILLS I MUST ACQUIRE _____
_____
_____
_____

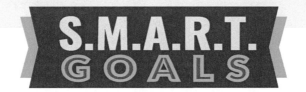

S.M.A.R.T. GOALS

SPECIFIC * MEASURABLE * ACTION-ORIENTED * REWARD-BASED * TIMELY

SHORT TERM GOALS	REWARDS
1.	1.
2.	2.
3.	3.

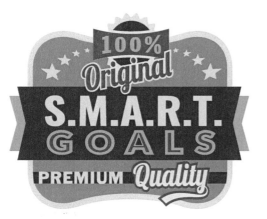

MY INSPIRATION PIC

[CHALLENGE 6] MAKE AN APPOINTMENT FOR FITNESS

If you ask the average woman on the street why she doesn't exercise regularly, the odds are the answer will be "I don't have time." The truth is, there isn't a single one of us who has enough time to do everything that needs to be done.

Most of the important "to dos" in our lives are scheduled in advance. Our calendars will reflect dentist, doctor, or hair stylist appointments, lunch with a friend, business meetings, play dates, and sports activities including games and practices for our children. Often missing from the calendar is time for "YOU" and your own fitness and health. Doesn't this deserve at least equal attention?

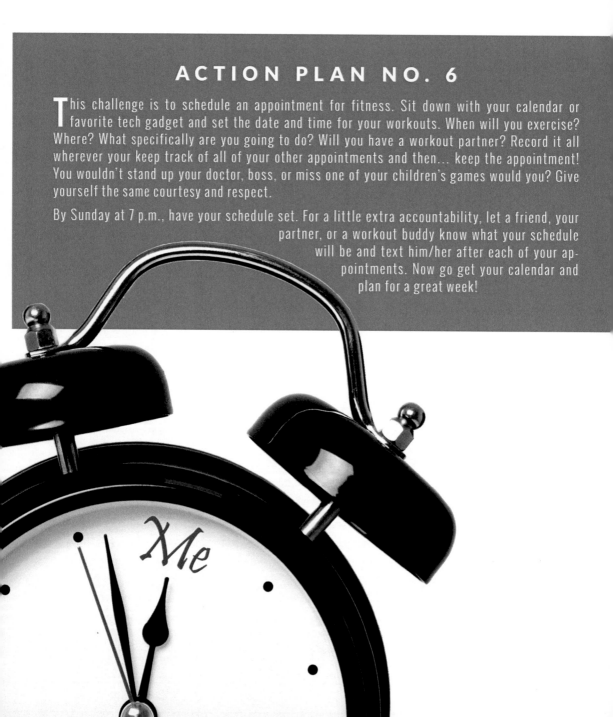

ACTION PLAN NO. 6

This challenge is to schedule an appointment for fitness. Sit down with your calendar or favorite tech gadget and set the date and time for your workouts. When will you exercise? Where? What specifically are you going to do? Will you have a workout partner? Record it all wherever your keep track of all of your other appointments and then… keep the appointment! You wouldn't stand up your doctor, boss, or miss one of your children's games would you? Give yourself the same courtesy and respect.

By Sunday at 7 p.m., have your schedule set. For a little extra accountability, let a friend, your partner, or a workout buddy know what your schedule will be and text him/her after each of your appointments. Now go get your calendar and plan for a great week!

[CHALLENGE 7] AVOID ISSUES WITH YOUR TISSUES

The last thing you want to have happen when you are finding your mojo is to be sidelined because of issues with your tissues. When I was younger, I always thought stretching was a waste of time and rest days were for "sissies." Learning to listen to my body, stretching, resting, and recovering is just as important as training.

I see this time and again with my mamas. Suzy is another classic example. She fell in love with bootcamp! She went from a life as a couch potato to training hard daily and rocking and rolling her mojo. Suzy had a clear goal and was focused on the prize. After a while, Suzy started having issues with her tissues, but continued to push through, not listening to her body. Her muscles were tight in her legs and lower back. Specifically, her knees were bothering her. Thinking "no pain; no gain" and not wanting to appear "whiny," she did not talk to her coach and continued to train. In essence, Suzy was overtraining by not taking time for recovery and stretching.

One day on a long run, she felt a "pop" in her knee. Fortunately for Suzy, her doctor diagnosed a stressed IT (Iliotibial) band and she was only sidelined for a few weeks. The last place she ever wanted to be was back on the couch, especially after finding her mojo. Had Suzy known that recovery and stretching is just as important as training, she could have avoided the injury and her downtime.

LEARN TO LISTEN TO YOUR BODY FOR SIGNS OF OVER-TRAINING. THIS MIGHT INCLUDE:

IRRITABILITY	PROLONGED MUSCLE SORENESS (OVER 72 HOURS)
SLEEPLESSNESS	
NOT RECOVERING FROM WORKOUTS	COMPROMISED IMMUNE SYSTEM
DIMINISHED PERFORMANCE DURING WORKOUTS	INCREASED CHANCE OF INJURIES
	DECREASED MOTIVATION
ELEVATED RESTING HEART RATE UPON WAKING	

If you experience one or more of these signs, you should allow time in your schedule for some R & R (rest and recovery). Minimally, you should take one day a week off to refresh your body and your mind. This includes adequate sleep (Challenge No. 34), hydration (Challenge No. 26), and stellar nutrition (see challenges in March, June, September).

Stretching is just as important as exercise. It improves your flexibility, your posture, and your blood flow. Increased blood and nutrient supply to muscle reduces soreness and increases your recovery. The bottom line is to use stretching to unwind your muscles for 10 minutes daily.

FLEXIBILITY STRETCHES

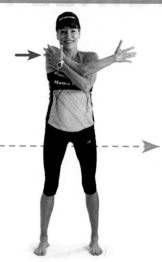

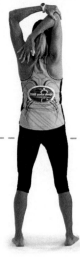

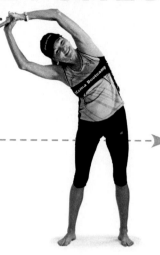

1. SHOULDER STRETCH
[SUPRASPINATUS STRETCH]
Keep your elbow parallel to ground.*

2. TRICEPS STRETCH
Pull elbow across and down.*

3. SIDE STRETCH
[LATERAL FLEXION STRETCH]
Exhale as you stretch outward.*

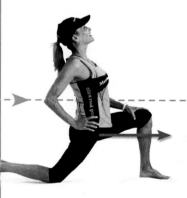

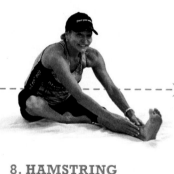

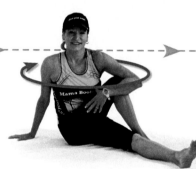

7. RUNNER'S STRETCH
[HIP FLEXOR STRETCH]
Keep back straight, tuck bottom under, lunge forward on front leg.*

8. HAMSTRING STRETCH
Knee slightly bent, gently straighten and reach for ankle.*

9. CROSS LEG STRETCH
[HIP ABDUCTOR STRETCH]
Cross leg over knee, look over opposite shoulder while pushing on knee with elbow.*

13.COBRA STRETCH
[LYING ABDOMINAL OR BHUJANGASANA STRETCH]
Do not overarch neck or back.

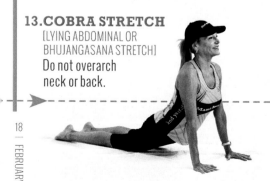

14.CHILD'S POSE
[LATISSIMUS DORSI STRETCH]
Sink into floor, with legs outside of torso. Breathe out as sinking down.

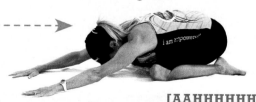

[AAHHHHHH!]

*DO ON BOTH SIDES OF BODY.

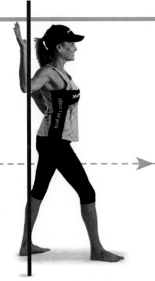

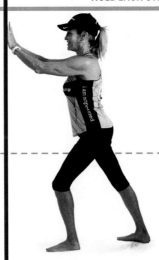

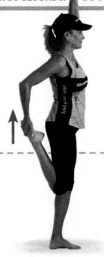

4. CHEST STRETCH
[PECTORALIS MAJOR STRETCH]
Rotate body away from wall or forward from pole.*

5. UPPER CALF STRETCH
[GASTROCNEMIUS STRETCH]
Hands on wall, back leg straight. Lean forward.*

6. STANDING QUAD STRETCH
[QUADROCEPS STRETCH]
Gently pull heel up and back to buttocks.*

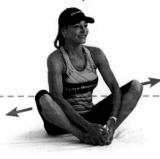

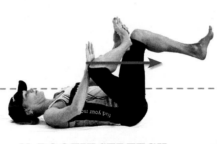

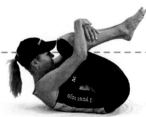

10. INNER THIGH STRETCH
[INNER THIGH HIP ADDUCTOR STRETCH]
Gently push knees toward floor. Keep back straight.

11. BOOTIE STRETCH
[GLUTIAL STRETCH]
Place foot above opposite knee. Lift leg towards chest, pressing on other knee.*

12. KNEE ROLL-IN/ LOWER BACK STRETCH
[LUMBAR FLEXION WITH ROTATION STRETCH]
Gently rock side-to-side.

ACTION PLAN NO. 7

Schedule a time and place for stretching daily. Is it after you get out of the shower in the morning? Is it at night while you are watching your favorite show? Is it during lunch while listening to music in your office? The point being is for you to schedule stretching into your day. Establish a routine so it becomes just like brushing your teeth, after all you wouldn't skip a day of brushing your teeth, right?!

If you take care of your body, it will take care of you. Hold each stretch 30 to 60 seconds and take 5 to 15 minutes to enjoy the process, paying particular attention to muscles that are tight. Breathe into the stretch and hold with no bouncing, pushing to the point of mild discomfort without pain.

[CHALLENGE 8] EXPRESS WORKOUT

Amy was a smoker and she was 110 pounds overweight. She worked in childcare at a minimum wage job. She was a single parent with a beautiful daughter. The father was MIA and she had a deadbeat boyfriend to boot. Not a pretty picture. One day Amy decided she was "sick and tired of being sick and tired" and she literally changed her mind.

She was ready for a change and cut out all soda. In only five weeks, Amy was surprised she dropped 26 pounds! Amy was ready to step up her game and needed more guidance to keep the momentum going. Asking her parents for help, they gave her 12 weeks of Mama Bootcamp as a Christmas gift. She started training and quit smoking. As Amy lost more weight, she gained more confidence. She decided to go back to school and eventually earned her bachelor's degree!

Being a single parent, working and going to school, exercise was not easy to fit into her tight schedule. To supplement her crazy, busy schedule and still squeeze in exercise time, I taught her about "Express Workouts." Consistency was the key. Amy found 15 minute blocks to get her workout completed three times weekly. BAM! Success was hers! Amy found her mojo: she lost over 110 pounds, broke up with the deadbeat boyfriend and found her confidence and strength.

One of the key components to building a healthy metabolic rate and your best body is increasing your lean muscle mass. The best way to do this is through strength training at least three times a week for a minimum of 15 minutes. The magic number is three. Two days of strength training a week is enough for maintenance, but at three times a week you will build lean muscle. Strength training can be done with free weights, bands, medicine balls, etc. or just your own body weight. What makes the "Express Workouts" so fantastic is that they do not require anything. You do not need a gym membership or special equipment, just you!

ACTION PLAN NO. 8

Rotate the three Express Workouts on a weekly basis. Put them on your calendar, and then honor yourself by doing them. If you need an accountability buddy, get one. No excuses. It is only 15 minutes. Studies show that short consistent, more frequent workouts, are better than one big workout a week to get results. No weights or equipment are required. Express workouts are great for travel, too.

Make a copy (or snap a pic) to take with you on the go!

BEGINNER EXPRESS WORKOUT

[CENTER PLANK] **30 seconds,** draw in abs

[ROLL-UP/ROLL-OUT] **20 repetitions**

[SIDE REACH] **20 repetitions** on right side, then **20 repetitions** on left side

[FLUTTER KICKS] **2 repetitions** of flutter kick 15 seconds / hold 10 seconds

[BUTT BUMPS] **20 repetitions**

[WALL SIT] **30 seconds**

AT LEAST THREE TIMES A WEEK FOR A MINIMUM OF 15 MINUTES

INTERMEDIATE EXPRESS WORKOUT

[CENTER PLANK] **45 seconds,** draw in abs

[ROLL-UP/ROLL-OUT] **25 repetitions**

[SIDE REACH] **25 repetitions** on right side, then **25 repetitions** on left side

[FLUTTER KICKS] **3 repetitions** of flutter kick 15 seconds / hold 10 seconds

[BUTT BUMPS] **25 repetitions**

[WALL SIT] **45 seconds**

AT LEAST THREE TIMES A WEEK FOR A MINIMUM OF 15 MINUTES

ADVANCED EXPRESS WORKOUT

[CENTER PLANK] **60 seconds,** draw in abs

[ROLL-UP/ROLL-OUT] **30 repetitions**

[SIDE REACH] **30 repetitions** on right side, then **30 repetitions** on left side

[FLUTTER KICKS] **4 repetitions** of flutter kick 15 seconds / hold 10 seconds

[BUTT BUMPS] **30 repetitions**

[WALL SIT] **60 seconds**

AT LEAST THREE TIMES A WEEK FOR A MINIMUM OF 15 MINUTES

EXPRESS WORKOUTS

PLANKING
30 SECONDS working up to **60 SECONDS**

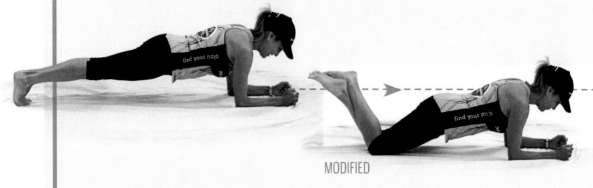

MODIFIED

SIDE REACHES
ON EACH SIDE
   beginner: **20 REPS**
   intermediate: **25 REPS**
   advanced: **30 REPS**

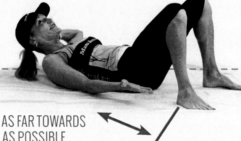

REACHING AS FAR TOWARDS
ANKLE AS POSSIBLE

BUTT BUMPS
   beginner: **20 REPS**
   intermediate: **25 REPS**
   advanced: **30 REPS**

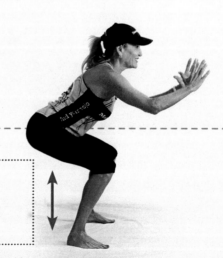

Bump up and down over
a real or imaginary seat,
going as low as possible.

REPEAT ENTIRE CIRCUIT **TWO** TO **FOUR TIMES**.

THINK YOU DON'T HAVE TIME TO EXERCISE? GUESS AGAIN! IN JUST 10 TO 20 MINUTES, YOU CAN GET AN EXCELLENT FULL BODY WORKOUT. YOU CAN DO IT WHEREVER YOU ARE AND WHENEVER YOU WANT! FOR A QUICK WORKOUT AT HOME, ON VACATION, OR EVEN IN THE OFFICE, TRY THIS SERIES OF EXERCISES.

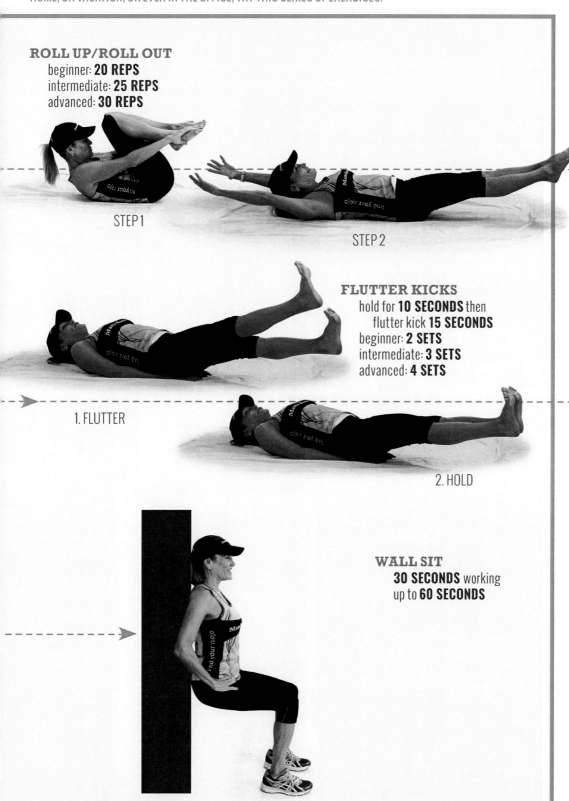

ROLL UP/ROLL OUT
beginner: **20 REPS**
intermediate: **25 REPS**
advanced: **30 REPS**

STEP 1

STEP 2

FLUTTER KICKS
hold for **10 SECONDS** then
flutter kick **15 SECONDS**
beginner: **2 SETS**
intermediate: **3 SETS**
advanced: **4 SETS**

1. FLUTTER

2. HOLD

WALL SIT
30 SECONDS working
up to **60 SECONDS**

FEBRUARY IN REVIEW

FOR FEBRUARY
MY GOALS

FOR FEBRUARY
MY GRATITUDE LIST

FOR FEBRUARY
RELATIONSHIPS TO INVEST IN

FOR FEBRUARY
WHAT'S GOING WELL

FOR FEBRUARY
WHAT NEEDS TO CHANGE

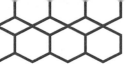

FEBRUARY NOTES

MY DOODLE SQUARE

MARCH

NUTRITION: SIMPLY EXPLAINED

IF YOU EAT LIKE CRAP, YOU WILL FEEL LIKE !#*@#!!.

NUTRITION STARTS WITH CLEAN EATING. CLEAN EATING, SIMPLY EXPLAINED, IS THE EATING OF HEALTHY, WHOLE, UNPROCESSED FOODS. AVOID PROCESSED FOODS - ANYTHING IN A BOX, BAG, CAN, OR PACKAGE, AND ALTHOUGH THERE ARE ALWAYS A FEW EXCEPTIONS TO THE RULE (LIKE A BAG OF FRESH GREEN BEANS), THE MAJORITY OF YOUR FOODS SHOULD BE FRESH. AVOID REFINED SUGAR.

FUELING YOUR BODY FOR RECOVERY, ENERGY AND HEALTH IS EQUALLY IMPORTANT AS EXERCISE. IN THE HEALTH AND FITNESS WORLD, THE "LAW OF THERMODYNAMICS" MEANS "CALORIES IN" (EATING) VS. "CALORIES OUT" (BURNING). IN ORDER TO LOSE WEIGHT, YOU NEED TO CREATE A DEFICIT.

I HAD A MAMA ("TINA") WHO ACTUALLY GAINED WEIGHT WHILE TRAINING FOR A MARATHON! SHE WOULD DO HER CORE EXERCISES, STRENGTH TRAINING AND SHORTER RUNS DURING THE WEEK AND LONG RUNS (10 PLUS MILES) ON THE WEEKENDS BURNING 1,000 – 2,000 CALORIES IN A SINGLE TRAINING. TINA WOULD THEN STOP BY HER FAVORITE BAGEL SHOP ON HER WAY HOME AND EAT TWO BAGELS WITH CREAM CHEESE (800-1,000 CALORIES EACH). SHE WAS EATING MORE CALORIES THAN SHE WAS BURNING THINKING SHE "EARNED" THOSE BAGELS, NOT REALIZING SHE WAS "SELF-SABOTAGING".

I NOT ONLY WANT YOU TO BE AT YOUR OPTIMAL WEIGHT, BUT ALSO TO HAVE A BEAUTIFUL "LEAN, MEAN, CALORIE BURNING MACHINE" WITH LOTS OF SLEEK DEFINED MUSCLE. NOT ONLY WILL EATING CLEAN GIVE YOUR BODY A METABOLIC BOOST, BUT IT WILL ALSO GIVE A CONFIDENCE BOOST! ATTITUDE AND ENERGY GO HAND IN HAND.

[CHALLENGE 9] GREEN SMOOTHIE

If I told you I could give you a pill that was anti-aging, anti-cancer, lowers your cholestrerol and blood pressure, stabilizes your blood sugar and strengthens your immune system, heals your body from the inside out with no side effects, you would jump on it right away. Especially if you heard it was reasonably priced and convenient to purchase, correct?

Well it is!! Experience the amazing results of drinking a green smoothie a day. Chock full of vitamins, minerals, chlorophyll, phyto-nutrients, fiber, and antioxidants, a daily dose of greens is the answer to a lot of common ailments. Here is a super simple chart to help you decipher how to make these magical concoctions. Out of all the challenges, I encourage you to turn this challenge into a daily lifestyle change.

SMOOTHIE CHART

GREENS }	KALE CHARD SPINACH	CELERY ARUGULA DANDELION	BROCCOLI PARSLEY CUCUMBER	WATERCRESS CILANTRO
FRUIT }	BANANAS APPLES ORANGES	MANGOES PINEAPPLE GUAVA	WATERMELON CANTALOUPE BLUEBERRIES	BLACKBERRIES STRAWBERRIES RASPBERRIES
LIQUID }	WATER COCONUT WATER	ALMOND MILK COCONUT MILK	CRANBERRY JUICE PEARS	
OPTIONAL & ADD-INS }	ROOT VEGES: CARROTS BEETS GINGER TURMERIC	ADD-INS: NUT BUTTERS PEANUT OR ALMOND	HEMP SEED FLAX SEED CHIA SEED	

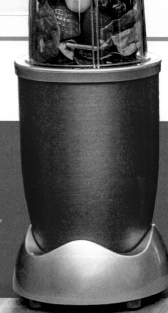

One last win/win for green smoothies: They are detoxing, healing, cleansing, energizing and one of the simplest most impactful things you can do daily to increase your quality of life.

ACTION PLAN NO. 9

Get your ingredients. Shop your local farmer's markets and fruit stands. In a hurry? There are many wonderful pre-packaged organic greens available in your grocery store. Purchase frozen fruit, or freeze your own. Pre-make your smoothie in a Nutri-Bullet™ (or similar processor) the day before and leave in your fridge. Blend when you are ready, add a straw and enjoy!

ACTION PLAN NO. 10

Close your kitchen right after dinner! Your body will love you for it!

[CHALLENGE 10]
CLOSE THE KITCHEN!

Late night snacking can sneak up on you when you don't even see it coming. That last bite of something left on the kitchen counter, a few cookies during the evening news, a cup of hot chocolate... Because you are slowing down for the day, late night calories don't get burned off. Instead, they go to bed with you, stowed away as fat.

To avoid late night munching, try "shutting down your kitchen" right after dinner.

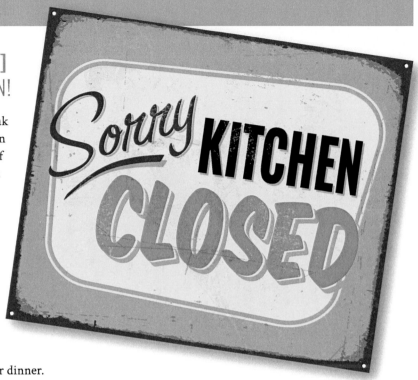

SHUT DOWN THE KITCHEN!

✓ PUT AWAY LEFTOVERS AND DO THE DISHES
✓ WIPE DOWN THE COUNTERS
✓ CLOSE THE BLINDS AND TURN OFF THE LIGHTS
✓ ONCE THE KITCHEN IS CLOSED, BRUSH YOUR TEETH.
   THIS WILL FURTHER DISCOURAGE YOU FROM SNACKING!

Creating a simple evening ritual of closing the kitchen can help you to avoid excess calories and bring an organized end to busy days.

ACTION PLAN NO. 11

Eat an apple a day. When you do your grocery shopping, branch out and try more than one variety of apple. Pay attention to what your favorites are, and make this challenge a part of your regular eating routine throughout the year.

[CHALLENGE 11] AN APPLE A DAY

You know that old saying "An apple a day keeps the doctor away?" Turns out it might be more true than you thought!

Apples are the perfect snack food. They are crunchy, sweet (but not too sweet), delicious and chocked full of nutrition. Apples are low on the glycemic index, which helps stabilize your blood sugar. They are also high in fiber which is not only good for your digestive system, but also helps you feel satisfied.

As an extra bonus, apples don't need to be refrigerated and come in their own "wrapping", making them the epitome of a "grab and go" snack.

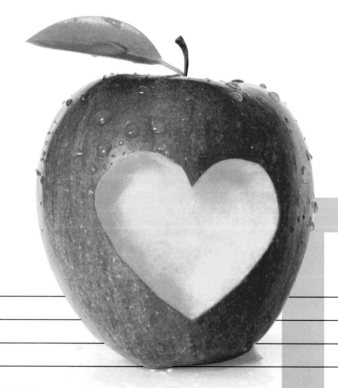

MAKE A LIST!
MY FAVORITE FOODS
TO PUT IN GRAB 'N GO'S...

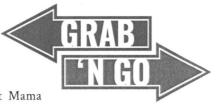

[CHALLENGE 12]

One of the cornerstones in our nutrition training at Mama Bootcamp is eating veggies. Lots and lots and lots of veggies.

You'd have to have been living under a rock to *not* know that a healthy diet must include lots of vegetables. But let's get real - even though we all *know* it, we don't all *do* it every day. For me, a big factor is the time – those veggies have to be washed, dried, and cut before I can eat them!

The small time investment is more than made up for by the benefit. By eating your veggies, you are not only loading yourself up with vitamins and minerals that are essential to healthy living, you are giving yourself so much more. Veggies not only help your body function better, but they can help you lose weight, look younger and even help prevent cancer. Sounds like a good deal to me!

Your challenge this week looks (and sounds familiar): Eat your veggies! But this week, let's work on making it part of your regular routine and making it *easy* (and fast, too!). You should be eating 10-12 servings of veggies every single day. With one serving the equivalent of a half of a cup, you can fit a whole day's worth of these health-making beauties into one quart-size plastic bag. We call these our "Grab 'N Go's".

Pick out several different veggies, and try to be sure to cover as many "colors" as you can. Dark green, light green and red are my favorites, with a little white thrown in, too. Chop them up into the size you

like best, and fill up your quart-sized bags. Put them in the fridge so they're ready to go (maybe pair them up with your favorite dip - hummus is mine).

With just a small time investment, the "work" is done for the whole week! On your way out door every morning, you can grab a bag full of yum! Snack on it all day long, and enjoy the awesome results.

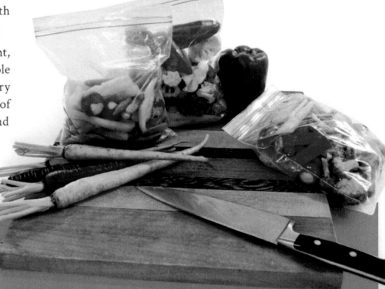

ACTION PLAN NO. 12

Shop on Saturday, prep on Sunday. The time and energy it takes to shop, wash, chop and bag your Grab 'N Go's can be overwhelming. I have found it much easier to shop on Saturday, and then prep on Sunday. Very doable without draining you. Use either eco-friendly Tupperware or quart sized Ziploc bags.

Whichever you choose, don't overthink it. Keep it simple and make it a weekend habit so you are ready to go when Monday comes.

MARCH IN REVIEW

FOR MARCH
MY GOALS

FOR MARCH
MY GRATITUDE LIST

FOR MARCH
RELATIONSHIPS TO INVEST IN

FOR MARCH
WHAT'S GOING WELL

FOR MARCH
WHAT NEEDS TO CHANGE

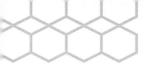

MARCH NOTES

_____
_____
_____
_____
_____
_____
_____
_____
_____
_____
_____
_____
_____
_____
_____
_____
_____
_____
_____
_____
_____
_____
_____
_____
_____

MY DOODLE SQUARE

APRIL

LIFE COACHING: CREATING A LIFE YOU LOVE

I LEARNED THAT WHAT YOU TALK ABOUT DEFINITELY COMES ABOUT. WHETHER YOU ARE COMPLAINING ABOUT YOUR THIGHS OR HATING YOUR JOB, THIS SORT OF TALK JUST KEEPS YOU STUCK.

SPRING IS ABOUT NEW BEGINNINGS AND FRESH STARTS. LET'S STOP WORDING OURSELVES INTO A PLACE WE DON'T WANT TO BE AND START CREATING A LIFE WE LOVE.

AND WOW, DID I LEARN THIS FIRST HAND. LET ME SHARE A STORY: I WAS RUNNING AROUND COMPLAINING ABOUT HOW LITTLE TIME I HAD WHILE STRUGGLING TO CREATE MORE. I WAS MULTITASKING WHENEVER I COULD. I WAS VERY UPSET WHEN MY PHONE DIED AND I WAS TOLD IT WOULD TAKE HOURS TO DOWNLOAD MY INFORMATION FROM "THE CLOUD." I IMMEDIATELY THOUGHT, "WHERE IS THIS CLOUD?" AND "WHY, IF WE'RE SO TECHNICALLY ADVANCED, IS IT GOING TO TAKE SO LONG?"

NOT HAVING ANY CONTROL OVER THIS SITUATION, I DECIDED I NEEDED TO TAKE A POSITIVE ATTITUDE THAT EVERYTHING WOULD WORK OUT OKAY.

SO FINALLY, ALL MY INFORMATION WAS DOWNLOADED INTO MY NEW PHONE AND READY TO GO. I SPENT THE NEXT HOUR OR SO DOUBLE CHECKING MY NEW PHONE SETTINGS AND APPS, MAKING SURE EVERYTHING WAS THERE. I LOADED INSTAGRAM AND THE APP ASKED TWO SIMPLE QUESTIONS THAT I HAD NOT NOTICED BEFORE: ALL CONTACTS? ALL FACEBOOK FRIENDS? I SAID "YES" TO BOTH AND ALL OF A SUDDEN I TRIPLED MY FOLLOWING IN ONE TOUCH OF MY FINGER! WOO HOO AND A HALLELUJAH! I WAS JUMPING FOR JOY AS MY PHONE WAS PINGING AS I ADDED NEW FOLLOWERS!

IF MY PHONE WOULD NOT HAVE GONE AWRY, I WOULD HAVE NEVER TRIPLED MY FOLLOWING IN SOCIAL MEDIA, SO THIS WAS MY SILVER LINING. THERE CAN BE A "SILVER LINING" TO YOUR CLOUDS (NO, PUN INTENDED!).

[CHALLENGE 13] SNAP! SNAP! COMPLAINT FREE ZONE

In January, we talked about paying attention to the positive things in your life. This week's challenge is the same idea: Whatever you feed grows.

This week, let's continue to feed the positive by eliminating negative self-talk and words from your life.

How many times in a day do you engage in negative self-talk? "I can't do this!" "My hips are too wide!" "I'm too slow a runner!" And how often do you complain about other things? "My husband never puts his dirty clothes in the hamper!" "My mother-in-law calls too early in the morning!"

We all do it, and it can be a hard habit to break!

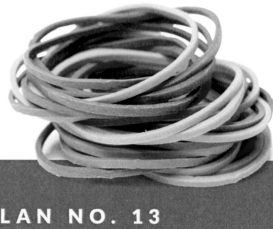

ACTION PLAN NO. 13

Purchase or find rubber bands that fit comfortably on your wrist (not too tight). Give yourself a little visual (and physical) reminder of this week's challenge. Put a rubber band around your wrist and wear it like a bracelet. When you catch yourself in a complaint or negative thought, give the band a tug. SNAP! SNAP! This will snap your train of thought right back to your new positive reality and break a bad habit. Additionally, it is much cheaper than therapy and very effective.

When you stop negatives thoughts, you have no choice but to focus on the positive. By feeding the positive, the good stuff grows and grows.

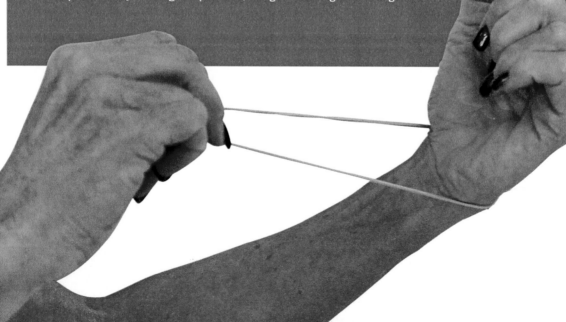

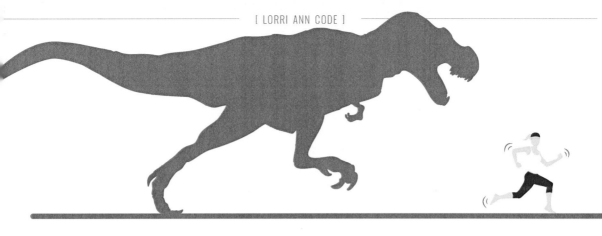

MOJO

Some motivation required.

[CHALLENGE 14] GET AND STAY MOTIVATED

motivation, *n.* [LL. *motivum, a moving cause*]

1. the act or process of giving someone a reason for doing something. the act or process of motivating someone. the condition of being eager to act or work.

2. a force or influence that causes someone to do something.

Here are two different scenarios: one motivated by fear and the second by hope.

FEAR. Mary came to Mama Bootcamp being on edge of full blown TYPE II diabetes. Her blood sugar was dangerously high. In addition, Mary was starting to have heart palpitations. Her mother had died of heart attack at the young age of 44 and Mary was turning 44 in the next month. She was very worried about the tolls her unhealthy lifestyle of stress, binge eating, and lack of exercise was taking on her body. Mary had heard about Mama Bootcamp for her co-worker, Kathy. Mary decided to go try a class on a free pass with Kathy after work one day. She was motivated by her fear of not wanting to repeat the health history of her mother.

HOPE. Susie had seen her best friend, Tina, join Mama Bootcamp. In a matter of a few months, Tina lost 24 pounds, dropped three pant sizes, and started training for a triathlon. Susie thought if Tina could do it, why couldn't she? She was motivated by hope for the future and thinking of the possibilities! Maybe she could train for a race and fall in love with exercise like her friend Tina!

These are both true stories and very real. Both Mamas were very motivated when they came to Mama Bootcamp! One was motivated by fear and the other by hope. Both very powerful motivators!

TIPS TO KEEP YOUR **MOJO MOTIVATION** ON **HIGH**

✓ Remind yourself of your goals by tracking your progress.

✓ Use your doctor's report as a baseline and schedule another appointment with him/her in six weeks.

✓ Post pictures of a scheduled event or location. Keep the invitation in a spot where you are reminded of "why?" you are working so hard. Hang the clothes you will be wearing at the event in plain site.

✓ Reward yourself for meeting your weekly check points. Check points are "in between" goals (also known as short term goals). Rewards, as you heard in Challenge #5, are very important for permanent change!

✓ Give yourself a break! Yes, you heard me right! Give yourself a few days off so you don't burn out. You want to keep your spirits and energy high! One of the best ways to do this is a planned break. You will come back motivated and ready to go! Make sure the break is not more than four days.

✓ Watch and read motivational stories or speeches. This will keep adding fuel to your fire! Inspiration is contagious so use it to your advantage by watching YouTube videos, reading stories that inspire you, and make sure you are sharing your goals with those that will cheer you on along the way.

✓ Eliminate distractions and time wasters. Limit yourself on Facebook, surfing the internet, or watching hours of television. Down time to "free" think is not a bad thing but give yourself time limits weekly, and then stick to them.

✓ "Fake it until you make it" is a cliché for a reason, because it works! Some days, you will not feel like working on your goals. Stay on task and do it any way. If after 30 minutes, you still are not feeling it, you still accomplished 30 minutes towards your goal!

✓ Surround yourself with people who are excited about life. Have you ever heard the saying "one bad apple, spoils the whole bunch?" Well, it is true! The same goes with people who are motivated, inspired, and enjoying life! Life is meant to be fun! Surround yourself with people who have similar values and energy.

ACTION PLAN NO. 14

In order to move forward, I want you to think about what motivates you. And then write it down to keep you moving!

Do you have an event you want to look your best for coming up? A wedding? Reunion? Vacation? Or did your doctor give you a serious warning or someone you care about have a life threatening event?

This year is all about "finding your mojo" and this challenge is so important to help you stay on track! Check in with what motivates you and go for it! Life can be exciting and full of adventure! But it won't feel that way if you are living life from the couch.

ACTION PLAN NO. 15

1. Make your To-Do list and put **YOU** at the top.
2. Say one nice thing about yourself every single day.
3. Bonus points for looking in the mirror and saying it!
4. Bonus, bonus points for writing it down and putting it where you can see it daily!
5. Do one nice thing for yourself. Reward yourself for just being.
6. Get a pedicure.
7. Plan a weekend getaway to someplace you want to go.
8. Find a new book to read.
9. Get a massage.

[CHALLENGE 15] DO UNTO YOU

The biggest challenge for women to remember when they are creating their "To-Do" list is to put themselves not just on the list, but at the top of the list. Does this make us bad mothers, wives, employees and friends if we are even on the list, let alone at the top? No.

I was raised to not think of "self." I was taught to be modest, stay quiet, and put others' needs before my own. As I grew wiser, I could see that this is a woman's disease, teaching us to become doormats and martyrs, and leading to unhealthy self-images.

Learning from my past experiences, and following the steps below, I was able to break out of an unhealthy cycle of being the doormat (among other things). How can we raise healthy, happy children, let alone be healthy and happy ourselves, if we are not recognizing and addressing our own physical, spiritual, and emotional needs?

We all have our own unique sets of circumstances, needs and expectations. Be true to yourself and discover what those are to you.

MAKE A LIST!
MY TO-DO LIST

* 1. Take Care of Me!
2.
3.
4.
5.

SPACES IN NEED OF DECLUTTERING...

ACTION PLAN NO. 16

This week, pick a drawer, a closet, or a room depending on your time and ambition and get rid of the junk! You can give away things you no longer use, and dust off the things you forgot you had! You will live more simply and freely as you declutter one step at a time.

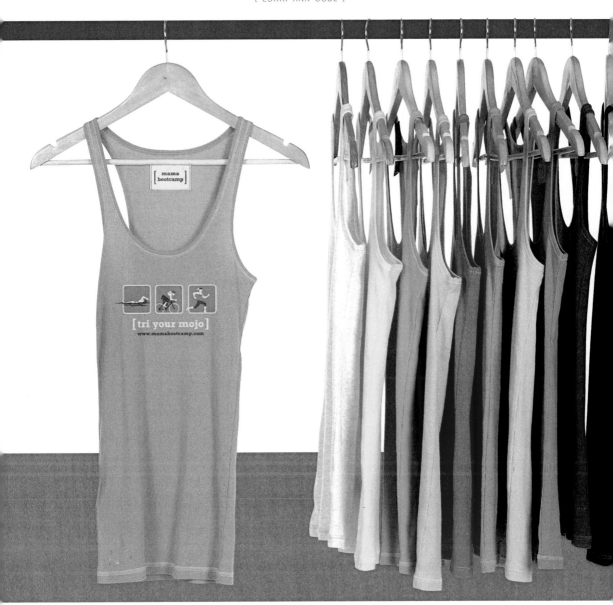

[CHALLENGE 16] DECLUTTER YOUR LIFE!

Clutter can be draining and de-energizing. By getting organized, you simplify and live a more meaningful life. I don't know about you, but when I'm surrounded by clutter, I have trouble focusing and getting things done. I am overwhelmed by "too much stuff" and cannot live my best life.

There are many tips and tools out there to get things organized in your home, office or car. What works for me is to keep it simple. A place for everything, and everything in its place. Stuff that I bring into my home that does not have a landing place very quickly becomes clutter.

As you move through your space, look for duplicates of things. Create a "donation" box and donate those duplicates to your favorite charity. Unburden yourself from things that can be replaced in the future.

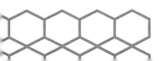

41 |

APRIL

FOR APRIL
MY GOALS

FOR APRIL
MY GRATITUDE LIST

FOR APRIL
RELATIONSHIPS TO INVEST IN

FOR APRIL
WHAT'S GOING WELL

FOR APRIL
WHAT NEEDS TO CHANGE

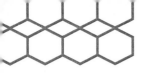

MY DOODLE SQUARE

MAY

FITNESS: NO ONE EVER DIED FROM THE BURN

[CHALLENGE 17]
SEXY, SENSATIONAL, SUPER SWIMSUIT CHALLENGE

[CHALLENGE18]
I'LL HAVE A SIDE OF BUTT/THIGHS WITH THAT, PLEASE!

[CHALLENGE 19]
BAM! BEAUTIFUL, BODACIOUS BACK AND ARMS

[CHALLENGE 20]
THE POWER OF THE PUSHUP

[CHALLENGE 21]
BFAS (BEAUTIFUL FABULOUS ARM SET!)

IT IS SUMMER TIME. VACATIONS AND SCHEDULES ARE ALL AWRY. SWIMSUITS, SHORTS AND TANK TOP SEASON IS HERE. TIME TO UP YOUR GAME. PICK ONE OF THESE CHALLENGES AND DO IT AT LEAST THREE DAYS A WEEK. OF COURSE, YOU CAN DO ALL OF THEM IF YOU ARE FEELING SUPER-MOTIVATED AND WANT TO CREATE THE TIME.

THIS NEXT TIP IS VERY IMPORTANT: DO YOU WANT TO RAISE YOUR METABOLIC RATE? STRENGTH TRAINING BUILDS LEAN MUSCLE MASS. MUSCLE BURNS MORE CALORIES THAN FAT. LOTS MORE!! FIVE POUNDS OF MUSCLE BURNS 350 CALORIES IN A DAY. THE SAME FIVE POUNDS OF FAT BURNS 30 CALORIES IN A DAY. LEAN MUSCLE IS YOUR CALORIE BURNING ENGINE AND RAISES YOUR METABOLIC RATE, EVEN WHILE YOU ARE SLEEPING!

MAKE SURE YOU EASE INTO STRENGTH TRAINING BY LISTENING TO YOUR BODY AND HONOR IT. BURNING IN YOUR MUSCLES IS GOOD. IT MEANS CHANGE IS HAPPENING. YOU ARE TEARING DOWN SMALL MUSCLE FIBERS, WHICH IN TURN WILL REBUILD BEAUTIFUL LEAN MUSCLE. GET FIRMER, TIGHTER, MORE TONED WITH THE FOLLOWING FUN AND QUICK EXERCISE CHALLENGES.

[CHALLENGE 17]
SEXY, SENSATIONAL, SUPER SWIMSUIT CHALLENGE

CORE WORKOUT

1. PLANKS: A. SIDE AND
Run through up to **4 REPS** per session.

B. CENTER [RIGHT AND LEFT]
Build up to **60 SECONDS EACH**

A.

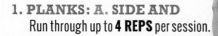
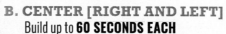

MODIFIED

B.

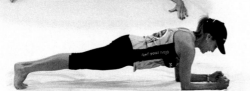
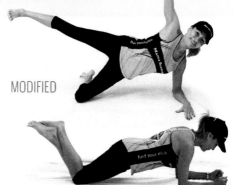

2. BICYCLES
30 REPS [count one side—no cheating!]

MODIFIED: TRICYCLE

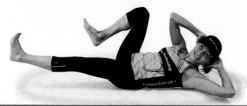
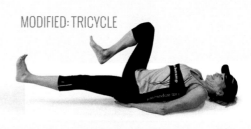

3. TORSO TWISTS
30 REPS

MODIFIED

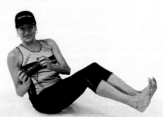
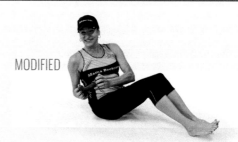

MODIFIED: ALTERNATE LIMBS

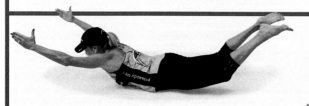
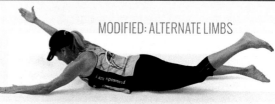

4. WONDER WOMAN
Run through up to **4 REPS** per session. Build up to **60 SECONDS EACH**

[CHALLENGE 18]
I'LL HAVE A SIDE OF BUTT/THIGHS WITH THAT, PLEASE!

BOOTY WORKOUT

RUN THROUGH THIS WORKOUT UP TO FOUR TIMES. START WITHOUT WEIGHTS AND ADD WEIGHTS AS YOU PROGRESS.

1. SQUATS
beginner: **20 REPS** or advanced: **30 REPS**

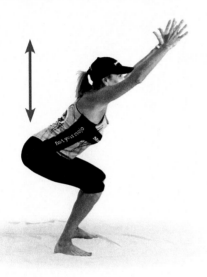

2. LUNGES
beginner: **20 REPS** or advanced: **30 REPS**

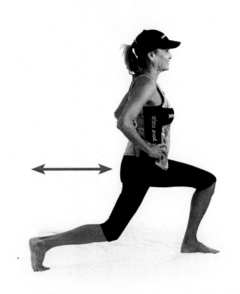

3. WALL SITS
Keep your core flexed.
beginner: **20 REPS** or advanced: **30 REPS**

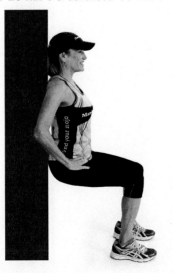

4. BUTT BLASTERS
beginner: **20 REPS** or advanced: **30 REPS**

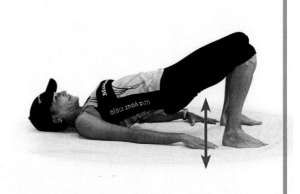

[CHALLENGE 19]
BAM! BEAUTIFUL, BODACIOUS BACK AND ARMS

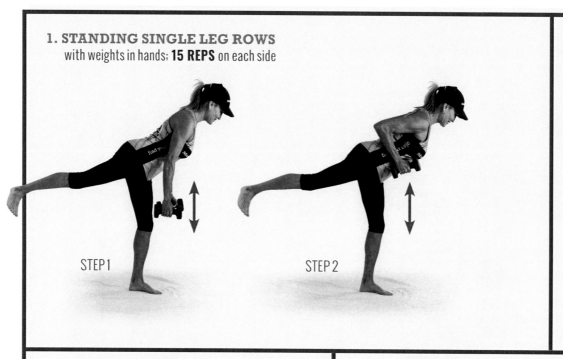

1. STANDING SINGLE LEG ROWS
with weights in hands; **15 REPS** on each side

STEP 1   STEP 2

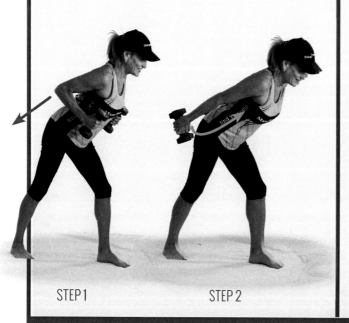

4. TRICEPS KICKBACKS
with weights in hands; **15 REPS** on each side

STEP 1   STEP 2

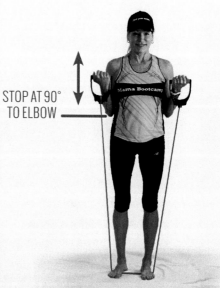

5. BICEP CURLS
15 REPS ON EACH SIDE
Use weights or band, your choice

STOP AT 90°
TO ELBOW

EQUIPMENT NEEDED: MEDIUM STRENGTH BAND WITH TWO HANDLES AND FIVE POUND WEIGHTS TO START WORKING YOUR WAY UP TO 15 POUND WEIGHTS.

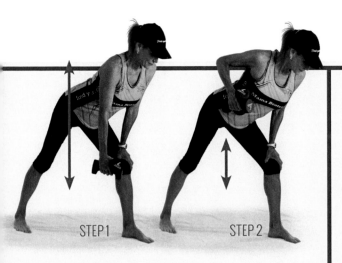

STEP 1

STEP 2

2. SINGLE ARM ROWS

with weight in hand: **10 REPS ON EACH SIDE.**
Double up the weight or use one heavier weight

3. SEATED ROW WITH BAND

one minute or **50 ROWS**
as a warm up

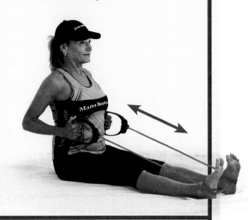

6. HAMMER CURLS

with weights in hands;
beginner: **20 REPS** or
advanced: **30 REPS**

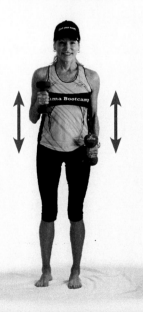

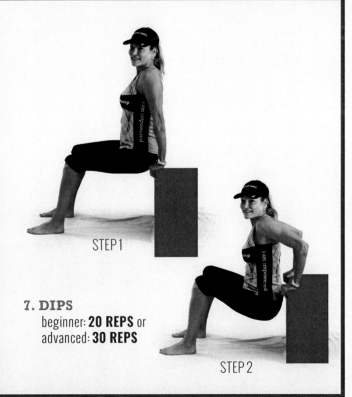

STEP 1

7. DIPS

beginner: **20 REPS** or
advanced: **30 REPS**

STEP 2

BAM! WORKOUT

[CHALLENGE 20] THE POWER OF THE PUSHUP

What do you do when you hear it's "time for pushups?" I'm willing to bet you groan, shoot a dirty look toward your trainer or, at a minimum roll your eyes. Admit it - you know it's true!

Pushups are not the easiest thing in the world to do. But they are worth every bit of effort you put into them. Pushups work *so* many muscle groups. Primarily, they work your deltoids (shoulders), triceps (back of the upper arm) and pectorals (chest). As if that weren't great enough, they can also engage your rhomboids (shoulder blade area), Erector spinae (muscles along your spine), rotator cuff, posterior deltoids (shoulders), serratus anterior (near your arm pits), rectus abdominus (abs), transverse abdominus (abs), gluteus maximus (buttocks), and quadriceps (thighs).

That's a lot of bang for your exercise buck, so it's no surprise they can be challenging!

Discover the power of the pushup! How many pushups can you do in one minute? Can you improve on that in one month? Do them whatever way works best for you - on your toes, on your knees, box style or even using a wall.

Challenge yourself to increase your strength and fitness with pushups. Your body will love you for it!

BOX PUSHUP
beginner: **20 REPS** or
advanced: **30 REPS**

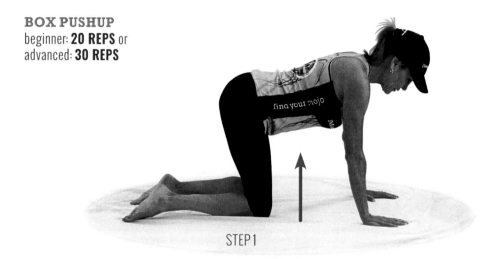

STEP 1

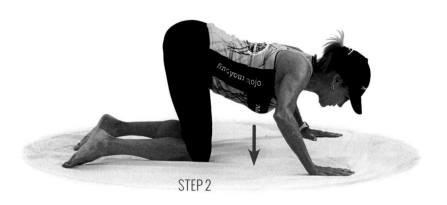

STEP 2

MODIFIED PUSHUP
beginner: **20 REPS** or
advanced: **30 REPS**

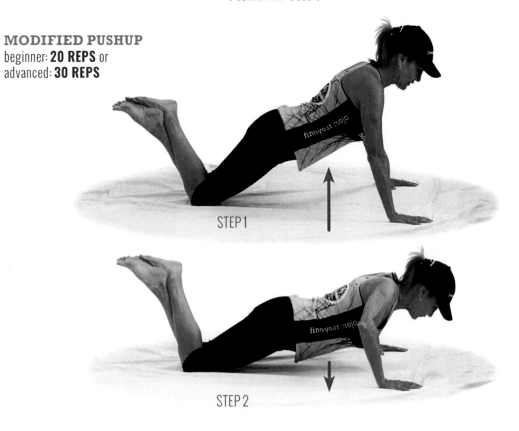

STEP 1

STEP 2

STANDARD PUSHUP
beginner: **20 REPS** or
advanced: **30 REPS**

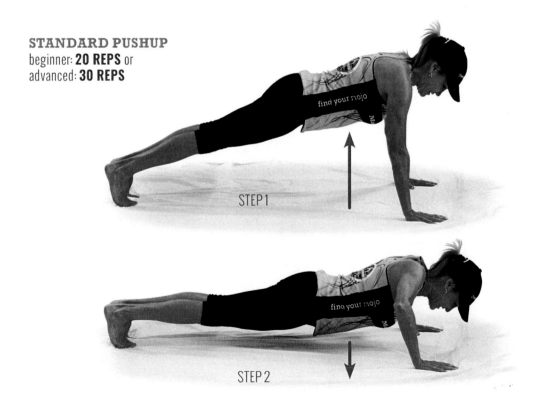

STEP 1

STEP 2

[CHALLENGE 21] BFAS (BEAUTIFUL FABULOUS ARM SET!)

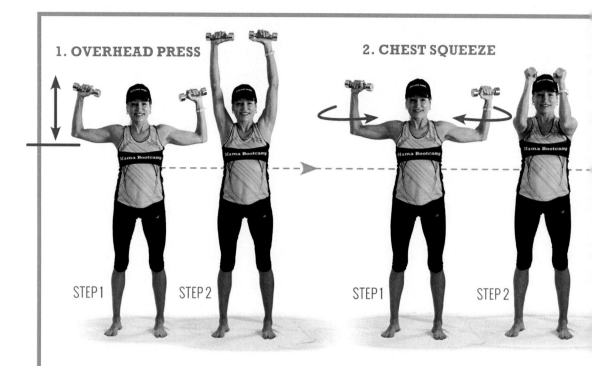

1. OVERHEAD PRESS

STEP 1   STEP 2

2. CHEST SQUEEZE

STEP 1   STEP 2

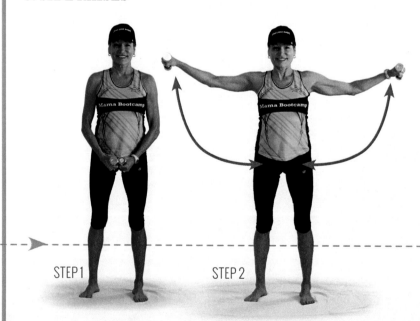

5. SIDE RAISES

STEP 1   STEP 2

10 REPETITIONS OF EACH EXERCISE.
REPEAT CIRCUIT **THREE TIMES**.

BEAUTIFUL

START OUT USING 3 TO 5 POUND WEIGHTS. DO NOT EXCEED 10 POUNDS PER WEIGHT. DO EXERCISES WITHOUT WEIGHTS IF YOU BECOME TOO FATIGUED.

3. BICEP CURLS

4. DOORKNOBS

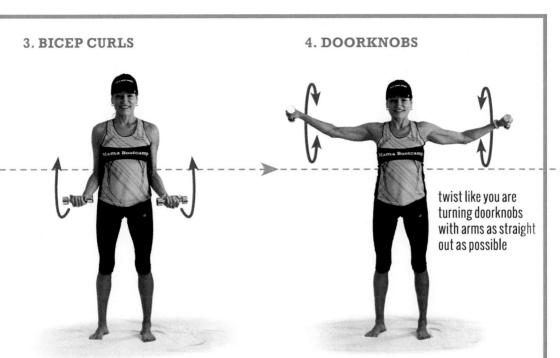

twist like you are turning doorknobs with arms as straight out as possible

6. TRICEP KICKBACKS

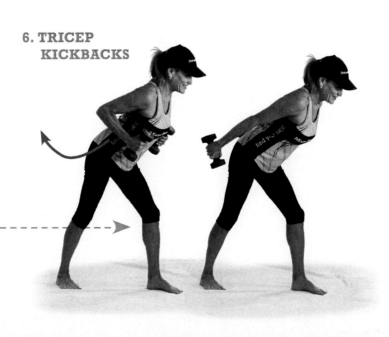

FABULOUS ARM SET

MAY IN REVIEW

FOR MAY
MY GOALS

FOR MAY
MY GRATITUDE LIST

FOR MAY
RELATIONSHIPS TO INVEST IN

FOR MAY
WHAT'S GOING WELL

FOR MAY
WHAT NEEDS TO CHANGE

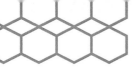

MAY NOTES

_____
_____
_____
_____
_____
_____
_____
_____
_____
_____
_____
_____
_____
_____
_____
_____
_____
_____
_____
_____

MY DOODLE SQUARE

_____
_____
_____
_____
_____

JUNE

NUTRITION:
KICK OUT THE "BRAIN FOG"

YOU ONLY HAVE ONE BODY IN LIFE. YOU PROBABLY HAVE NOT ALWAYS TREATED IT THE BEST. GROWING AND LEARNING IN LIFE INVARIABLY INCLUDES SOME ABUSE TO YOUR BODY, WHETHER IT IS TOO MUCH ALCOHOL, DRUGS (PRESCRIPTION OR OTHERWISE), SUGAR ADDICTION, OVER EATING, UNDER MOVING (AKA: BEING A COUCH POTATO), OVER STRESSED, AND EVEN YO-YOING ON CRAZY DIETS. ALL OF THESE ARE EXTREMELY HARSH ON YOUR BODY AND CAN CREATE "BRAIN FOG." IT IS HARD TO FIND YOUR MOJO WHEN YOU CANNOT THINK CLEARLY.

BEFORE WE MOVE ON, LET'S TALK A BIT ABOUT DIETS. WHAT ARE THE FIRST THREE LETTERS OF DIET? THAT'S RIGHT! D-I-E. THERE'S NOTHING GREAT ABOUT THAT!

DIETS DO NOT WORK FOR LONG TERM WEIGHT LOSS. SO LET'S STOP THE YO-YO DIETS. ALBERT EINSTEIN SAID THE DEFINITION OF INSANITY IS DOING THE SAME THING OVER AND OVER AND EXPECTING DIFFERENT RESULTS. LET'S GET OFF THAT ROLLER COASTER. LET'S AGREE TO CHANGE HOW WE THINK ABOUT FOOD AND DIETING AND KICK OUT THE "BRAIN FOG."

ONE OF THE MOST FRUSTRATING REALITIES OF DIETING IS THAT IF YOU CUT TOO MANY CALORIES, YOUR METABOLISM THINKS TIMES ARE LEAN. IT IS JUST THE OPPOSITE. IT PUTS THE BRAKES ON FAT-BURNING TO CONSERVE ENERGY. YOU NEED TO EAT ENOUGH CALORIES TO KEEP YOUR METABOLIC RATE ON HIGH.

IT IS HARD TO FEEL ENERGIZED, EXCITED, AND INVIGORATED IF YOU ARE EATING FOODS HIGH IN SATURATED FAT, SUGAR, SALT AND/OR DRINKING DAILY (ALCOHOL IS A DEPRESSANT, FOLKS). WHAT YOU EAT AND DRINK CAN HELP KICK THE "BRAIN FOG" OUT OF YOUR BODY, SO YOU CAN FEEL GREAT AND THINK WITH CLARITY.

CLEAN EATING IS AN IMPORTANT CONCEPT FOR KICKING OUT THE "BRAIN FOG." EATING CLEAN IS NOT ABOUT HOW WELL YOU WASH YOUR VEGETABLES. IT IS STRIVING TO EAT WHOLE UNPROCESSED FOODS AND LIMITING SALT, SUGAR, AND SATURATED FATS. THE LESS PROCESSED YOUR FOOD IS THE BETTER YOU WILL FEEL. READ THE LABEL. IF THE FIRST FEW INGREDIENTS ARE SUGAR (OR A DERIVATIVE) OR WORDS YOU CANNOT PRONOUNCE, PUT IT DOWN! THIS IS NOT A WHOLE FOOD; IN FACT IT MIGHT NOT BE FOOD AT ALL. JUNK FOOD IS CALLED "JUNK" FOR A REASON.

THE FOLLOWING CHALLENGES ARE SIMPLE. BUT THESE ARE AREAS THAT YOU WILL WANT TO LAYER ON ONE AT A TIME. IN ORDER TO MASTER EACH ONE, YOU MAY NEED MORE THAN ONE WEEK.

DAILY CLEAN EATING STRATEGY TO KICK OUT THE "BRAIN FOG"

✓ EAT 10 TO 12 SERVINGS OF FRESH ORGANIC FRUITS AND VEGETABLES PER DAY.

✓ DRINK 80 TO 100 OUNCES OF WATER A DAY.

✓ EAT LEAN PROTEIN WITH EVERY MEAL.

✓ LIMIT PROCESSED FOODS.

✓ EAT EVERY 2 TO 4 HOURS TO STABILIZE YOUR BLOOD SUGAR AND INCREASE YOUR ENERGY.

✓ DO NOT SKIP MEALS — NO STARVATION ALLOWED!

QUICK TIP LIMIT YOUR SHOPPING TO THE PERIMETER OF THE STORE. THINK ABOUT IT. ALL OF THE BOXED FOODS, CHIPS, CANDY, COOKIES, ETC. ARE IN THE MIDDLE OF THE STORE. YOUR FRESH PRODUCE, LEAN PROTEIN, DAIRY PRODUCTS ARE FOUND ON THE PERIMETER OF THE STORE.

BONUS! BONUS!

[CHALLENGE 22] BREAK YOUR FAST

You know that old saying "Breakfast is the most important meal of the day." It is an old saying for a reason — it is *true!*

It is hard to rock your mojo and feel energized if you are skipping breakfast. Breakfast literally means "breaking the fast." You probably have not eaten for 8-10 hours. To kick start your day and stabilize your blood sugar, you need breakfast. But somehow it seems to be the hardest meal for many people to eat. They don't want to eat in the morning or they are too busy.

Sure, you can start your day with a quick donut, croissant, sugar laden cereal or white chocolate mocha. You might as well mainline a syringe of sugar into your blood stream, because this breakfast will spike your blood sugar levels. By making these choices, you are starting your day without giving your body a fighting chance! Remember what goes up, must come down. Your sugar-infused blood levels spike and "bonk" (come crashing down) causing you to start your day in a cycle of highs and lows with your body trying to chase energy all day long.

Instead, start your day with a good dose of protein and complex carbohydrates. It will prevent the hills and valleys of blood sugar spikes and "bonks," keeping you energized and mentally clear.

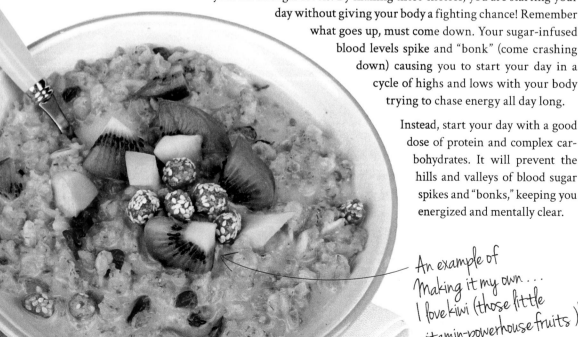

An example of making it my own . . . I love kiwi (those little vitamin-powerhouse fruits)!!!

ACTION PLAN NO. 22

Start **EVERY** day with a clean, healthy, nutrient-rich breakfast! Plan your breakfast with both carbohydrates and protein for great metabolism and energy. You might find, as I do, that starting the day eating clean makes it easier to eat right all day long!

BREAKFAST IDEAS

OATMEAL
EAT YOUR OATMEAL WITH A COUPLE OF SCRAMBLED EGG WHITES FOR ADDED PROTEIN
ADD INS: GROUND FLAX, CHIA SEEDS, CHOPPED NUTS, BERRIES, OTHER FRUITS
COOK YOUR OATMEAL IN ADVANCE AND FREEZE IT IN INDIVIDUAL-SIZE PORTIONS.
OATMEAL IS A WONDERFUL VEHICLE FOR NUTRITION.
STEEL-CUT OATS ARE MORE NATURAL AND NUTRITIOUS THAN INSTANT OATMEAL.

ONE HARD BOILED EGG
WITH WHOLE-GRAIN TOAST, NUT BUTTER AND FRUIT

ONE POACHED EGG
ON WHOLE-GRAIN TOAST WITH FRESH FRUIT

ONE SCRAMBLED EGG
WHOLE-GRAIN ENGLISH MUFFIN WITH LIGHT CREAM CHEESE, ONE SLICED APPLE
AND LOW-FAT OR SKIM MILK

PLAIN, FAT-FREE GREEK YOGURT
ADD INS: CHOPPED FRUIT, QUINOA, GRANOLA, NUTS
GREEK YOGURT HAS THE HIGHEST PROTEIN CONTENT OF ALL YOGURTS.

HIGH-FIBER, WHOLE GRAIN CEREAL
WITH LOW-FAT OR SKIM MILK AND FRESH FRUIT

WHOLE-GRAIN TOAST
TOP WITH 2 TABLESPOONS OF NUT BUTTER AND FRUIT SLICES

QUICK TIP:
EAT BREAKFAST LIKE A QUEEN,
LUNCH LIKE A PRINCESS,
AND DINNER LIKE A PAUPER.

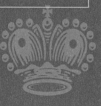

MOJO IN A JAR SALADS

LAYER IN THIS ORDER:	GREEK SALAD	MIXED GARDEN	SPINACH SALAD
1. DRESSING }	GREEK DRESSING	BALSAMIC VINAIGRETTE	RASPBERRY OR DIJON VINAIGRETTE
2. 'WET' VEGGIES }	OLIVES RED ONIONS CUCUMBER TOMATOES	SHREDDED CARROT PEPERONCINI SLICED SCALLIONS RED OR YELLOW BELL PEPPER	RED ONION MUSHROOMS SLICED PEAR
3. EXTRAS }	FETA CHEESE WALNUTS	PARMESAN CHEESE SUNFLOWER SEEDS	HARD BOILED EGG DRIED CHERRIES OR CRANBERRIES
4. GREENS }	ROMAINE LETTUCE OPTIONAL KALE OPTIONAL SPINACH	MIXED BABY GREENS OPTIONAL SPINACH OPTIONAL BABY HERB GREENS	SPINACH OPTIONAL KALE OPTIONAL CHARD

ACTION PLAN NO. 23

Set up your own schedule for shopping and preparing. Your goal is to have meals and snacks on hand so you do not have to run to your nearest fast food restaurant. Here are one of my favorite ideas to help you plan for your week...

Mojo in a Jar salads keep in the fridge for up to five days. Use a one quart wide-mouth mason jar. The key is to keep the dressing away from your greens, so layer your dressing on the bottom. Next, layer your wet vegetables. Then, place your extras and greens on the top and seal.

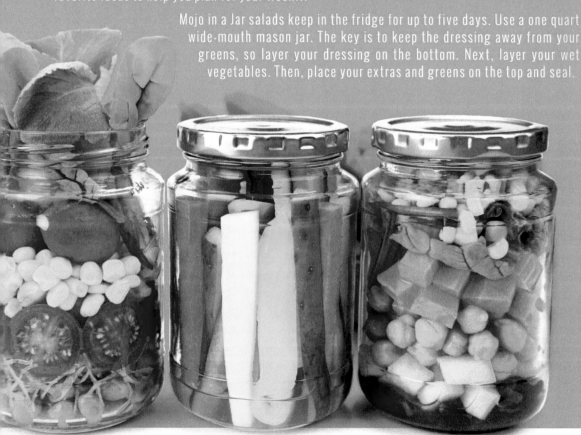

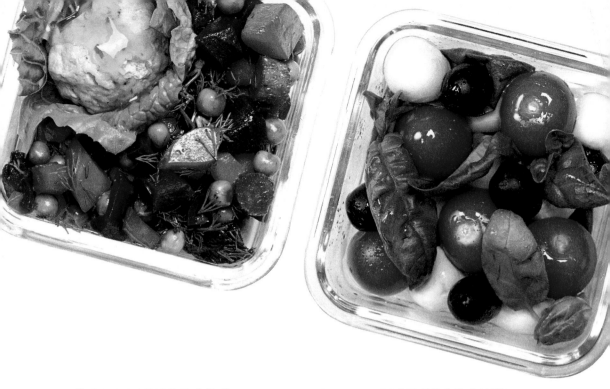

[CHALLENGE 23] STAY OUT OF THE FAST FOOD LINE

So there I am in line at the fast food restaurant, starving and wanting to eat *everything* on the menu. I know it will taste great going down, but literally "numb" me in about 15 minutes. I will end up feeling gross, bloated, and sluggish. There is nothing good about "fast food", whether it is at a restaurant or your local convenience store. After going through the cycles of gorging on fast food, I decided I was done.

I started prepping my own food with an emphasis on clean and healthy eating. Keeping it simple was, and is, very important in my life. I preplanned when I would shop, wash, cut, cook and/or bag my food. For me, my Saturdays are my "shopping" days and Sundays are my "prep" days.

MEAL IDEAS TO MAKE YOUR OWN 'CLEAN FAST FOOD'

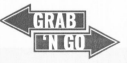

✓ GRAB 'N GO VEGGIE BAGS (see challenge 12, page 31)

✓ MOJO IN A JAR SALADS (previous page)

✓ NATURE'S WRAPPED FOODS: bananas, oranges, apples, etc.

✓ PROPORTIONED HEALTHY PROTEIN SNACKS: string cheese, nuts, yogurt

✓ BENTO BOX MEALS with protein, complex carbohydrates, and vegetables. You can use your leftovers to build these meals or prepare the ingredients on your prep day. Be sure to use all three food groups. Examples are:
>   Turkey meatball / sweet potatoes / green beans
>   Chicken / brown rice / broccoli, carrot & cauliflower medley

PREPLAN FOR A HAPPY, HEALTHY WEEK. THIS WILL KEEP YOU OUT OF THE FAST FOOD LINE, SAVING YOU TIME, MONEY AND BONUS, BONUS... YOU WILL FEEL GREAT!

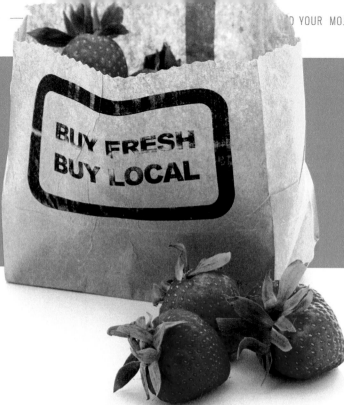

ACTION PLAN NO. 24

Eat **LOCAL** by shopping at a farmer's market near you or visit your local food co-op. Take a look around and choose food that is seasonal, local, delicious and healthy. Your body will love you for it!

[CHALLENGE 24]
EAT LOCAL!

You hear it all the time: Eat Local! But why? There are are many reasons to eat local foods…

Local foods are fresher and taste better.

Fresh locally harvested foods have their full, whole favors intact. Transportation, refrigeration, and being held in a warehouse for days all cuts the flavor of the food. Fresh food lasts longer, too.

Local foods are seasonal, with a greater variety available.

Local foods usually have less environmental impact.

Buying foods grown and raised near where you live helps maintain farmland and green space in your area and reduces transportation costs.

Local foods promote food safety.

The fewer steps there are between your food's source and your table the less chance there is of contamination. Also, local foods at your farmer's market are not treated with irradiation (using radiation to kill germs) and preservatives (such as wax) to protect the produce while traveling.

Local foods support your local economy and save you money.

Money spent with local farmers, growers, and locally-owned businesses all stays close to home, working to build your local economy instead of being handed over to a corporation in another city, state, or country. Since the food moves through fewer hands, more of the money you spend tends to get back to the people growing it.

Local foods create community.

Knowing where your food is from connects you to the people who raise and grow it. Instead of having a single relationship—to a big supermarket—you develop smaller connections to more food sources: vendors at the farmers' market, the local cheese shop, your favorite butcher, the co-op that sells local eggs, a local café that roasts coffee.

[CHALLENGE 25]
BECOME A LEAN, MEAN CALORIE-BURNING MACHINE

I sat down with a new mama, Beth, who was just starting Bootcamp. As we were doing her intake (initial consultation, goal-setting, measurements), I asked her what brought her to Bootcamp. In an angry tone of voice, Beth started to explain her frustrations. She was not losing weight in spite of her best efforts. She went on to say she started her day with coffee, not eating between meals, and only "occasionally" falling off the wagon and binge eating. Dinner was her only time with her husband. They sat down for a "nice" meal together at the end of the day. She shared that this was the ONLY time she really ate anything! Why couldn't she lose the weight?

Beth's confusion around how to eat is not uncommon. Growing up, a lot of us have heard the conventional, "three square meals a day with no snacking." Frequently, I hear women say," I skip breakfast, so I can save my calories for a big lunch or the party tonight!" Well this, my friends, is exactly how sumo wrestlers eat to gain as much fat as possible! They skip breakfast, do not snack between meals, and purposely wait six to eight hours between eating to trick their body into storing as much *fat* as possible! In fact, when your body thinks it is starving, it will use lean muscle for energy.

Muscle is your "calorie burning engine." Saving muscle and losing fat is the goal. By skipping breakfast and snacks, you are tricking your body into becoming cannibalistic, eating away at the "engine." No wonder Beth was frustrated. She was in training to be a *sumo wrestler!* It was definitely time for some education and information so Beth could get on the right track!

Another way to raise your metabolic rate is to eat frequently. If you do not eat often enough, your body goes into "starvation protection" mode, conserving calories, storing fat, and burning muscle (not fat) for energy. After four hours of fasting, your metabolism begins to slow down. By eating every two to four hours, you repeatedly reset your metabolism so it stays in high gear, and you burn fat all day long. Your metabolic rate (the lean, mean, calorie burning machine) needs to be fed in order to be healthy and strong. You will also curb your levels of cortisol — the "stress hormone" — and flatten your belly in the process. You will have more energy and less hunger, because eating every two to four hours keeps your blood sugar levels steady. This is the perfect recipe for finding your mojo!

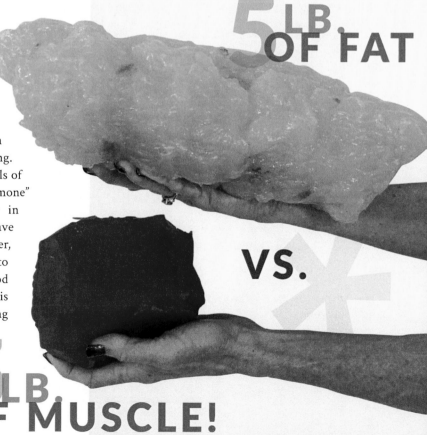

5 LB. OF FAT

VS.

5 LB. OF MUSCLE!

ACTION PLAN NO. 25

Eat frequently! Carry snacks with you, such as almonds, hard boiled eggs, apples, yogurt, bananas, oranges, cheese sticks, tuna kits with whole grain crackers, etc. The best snacks provide enough calories to be satisfying, but not so many that the snack becomes a meal. Choose snacks with whole grains, fiber, and/or protein as these give them staying power. I recommend keeping your snacks under 200 calories.

Kick start your day with breakfast. Breakfast is particularly important if you want to maximize your metabolic potential. When you are sleeping, your physical activity decreases, your breathing rate decreases and your heart rate decreases. Even if you eat before bed, your metabolism naturally slows because your energy requirements are lowered. Eating first thing in the morning, and not just coffee on an empty stomach, "kick-starts" your metabolism for the day. (See Challenge No. 23)

Preparing your snacks so you are ready to go is imperative! I try to plan for the season. For example, if it is the middle of summer, I make sure I have a larger size ice chest or insulated lunch pail. I keep mine next to the refrigerator on the counter. On early work mornings, it is there and ready to go. I have no reason to "forget" my snacks, salads, fresh fruit, etc. I also keep it packed with prepackaged almonds, bars, and my wrapped vitamins so **nothing** gets in the way of my mojo!

Make your lists of staples and include them on your grocery list. Mojo is serious business and I want you to make sure you are giving it all the attention it deserves!

[CHALLENGE 26] DRINK YOUR WATER

One of clients, Nancy, was very distracted during a training session. I asked Nancy what was wrong and she shared that her 15 year old son was suffering from severe headaches and they were taking him to the doctor for testing. I asked if he was drinking water. Nancy commented that he drank sodas all day long, but she could not remember the last time she'd seen him drink water. One of the first signs of dehydration is headaches. Nancy took away the soda and had him drink water. His headaches disappeared.

The third way to raise your metabolic rate is hydration. The first sign of dehydration is fatigue and the second sign is headaches. How can you find your mojo if you are feeling tired and just plain bad? Drinking water is one of the easiest ways to improve your health and change your body. I recommend you drink 80 – 100 ounces every single day.

OTHER THAN THE FACT THAT WATER TASTES REFRESHING AND CLEAN, THERE ARE SO MANY OTHER BENEFITS TO STAYING HYDRATED

WATER FACTS

Your body is over 80% water.

Being hydrated reduces/eliminates headaches and gives you energy.

Drinking water is an appetite suppressant. Most of the time that you think you are hungry you are actually thirsty.

WATER HELPS

Your kidneys function properly.

Your liver metabolize and flush out fat and toxins.

Your skin and hair by moisturizing from the inside out.

When you are 2 percent dehydrated you burn a full 30 percent less calories.

WATER CONSUMPTION TIMING

2 glasses of water after waking up helps activate internal organs.

1 glass of water 30 minutes before a meal helps digestion.

1 glass of water before taking a bath helps lower blood pressure.

1 glass of water before going to bed helps avoid stroke or heart attack.

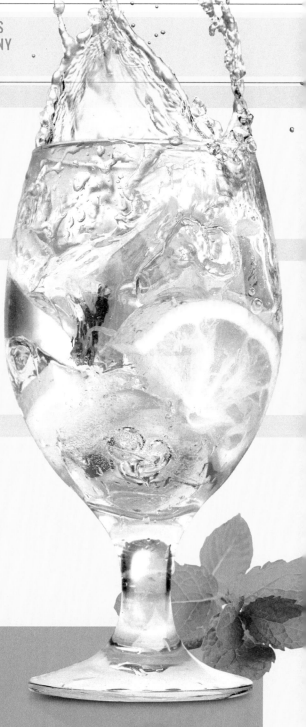

ACTION PLAN NO. 26

Let me give it to you straight. Drink 40 ounces of water by noon. Drink another 40 ounces of water by 6 pm. Anything after that is bonus, bonus. Make it happen by having 40 ounces sitting on your desk, ready to drink so you can track it. Find a favorite water bottle or glass if you are going to be eco-friendly and refill. If you are still having a hard time drinking your water, make your own spa water by adding slices of limes, lemons, oranges, cucumber or a pinch of mint. After all, you deserve it!

JUNE IN REVIEW

FOR JUNE
MY GOALS

FOR JUNE
MY GRATITUDE LIST

FOR JUNE
RELATIONSHIPS TO INVEST IN

FOR JUNE
WHAT'S GOING WELL

FOR JUNE
WHAT NEEDS TO CHANGE

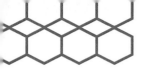

JUNE NOTES

(ruled note lines)

MY DOODLE SQUARE

JULY

LIFE COACHING:
FACE LIFE WITH STRENGTH AND GRACE

IT IS FUNNY WHEN I HEAR WOMEN SAY TO ME "OH, BUT YOU 'NEVER' EAT THAT" OR "YOU HAVE ALL THE TIME, MOTIVATION, EXPERTISE, COMMITMENT...BLAH, BLAH, BLAH, AND YOUR WORLD IS SO PERFECT, YOU CAN TRAIN ALL DAY LONG".

IT IS ASSUMED BECAUSE I AM A TRAINER, LIFE COACH, AND TRIATHLETE THAT I RARELY HAVE ANY CHALLENGES WITH TIME, TRAINING, FOOD, SLEEP, AND GOD FORBID... MOTIVATION!

WELL, I AM HUMAN AND I AM ALWAYS TRYING TO FIND BALANCE BETWEEN MY KIDS (WHO NEED ME JUST AS MUCH NOW), MY HUBBY (WHO I ACTUALLY LOVE TO SPEND TIME WITH), MY CAREER (WHICH IS MY PATH, PASSION AND JOY), MY OWN TRAINING AND RACING, AND MY SLEEP (WHICH GENERALLY SUFFERS FIRST). I FIND MYSELF BEING PULLED IN A LOT OF DIFFERENT DIRECTIONS DAILY; THIS IS A CHALLENGE FOR ME. I OFTEN SAY TO MY COACHES: "A TEACHER (COACH) IS ALWAYS TEACHING WHAT SHE NEEDS TO LEARN HERSELF." YES, IT IS TRUE... I AM. HERE ARE TWO THINGS I KNOW FOR SURE THAT I CAN SHARE WITH YOU:

I AM THANKFUL THAT I HAVE SURROUNDED MYSELF WITH AMAZING, STRONG WOMEN; WOMEN WHO WANT TO LIVE GOOD LIVES, AS DRAMA-FREE AS POSSIBLE. THESE ARE WOMEN I TRAIN WITH, WORK WITH, CRY WITH, VENT WITH, LAUGH WITH AND "FIGURE THINGS OUT" WITH. HAVING A STRONG CIRCLE OF PEOPLE WHO LOVE YOU AND SUPPORT YOU WHEN THE CHIPS ARE DOWN IS A LIFE CHANGER. I HAVE NOT ALWAYS HAD THIS AND I CAN TELL YOU... IT IS ONE OF THE SECRETS TO A GREAT LIFE.

IT IS NOT WHAT HAPPENS TO YOU IN LIFE, BECAUSE "STUFF" WILL ALWAYS HAPPEN, BUT INSTEAD HOW YOU HANDLE IT. MOVING THROUGH CHALLENGES, DISAPPOINTMENTS AND TRAUMAS WITH GRACE AND COURAGE BUILDS CHARACTER, STRENGTH AND INTEGRITY. WHEN YOU FACE A PROBLEM, IT BUILDS YOUR SENSE OF SELF. GIVING UP WHEN IT GETS TOUGH IS DEMORALIZING AND DISCOURAGING; IT CAN ALSO TAKE A PRETTY BIG CHUNK OF YOUR SELF-CONFIDENCE. TRY, AND IF YOU FAIL, GET BACK UP AND TRY AGAIN! "DO-OVERS" ARE A BEAUTIFUL THING.

MAY THIS MONTH'S CHALLENGES HELP YOU MOVE THROUGH LIFE WITH STRENGTH AND GRACE.

[CHALLENGE 27] ELIMINATE THE FRENEMIES

In Challenge 16, you picked a physical area to declutter in your life. My mamas have shared their de-cluttering stories about their cars, closets, and even refrigerators! Don't you love the freeing feeling of getting rid of the junk that was draining you of your energy and your time? Well, this is a decluttering of the spirit. An emotional kind of clean-up.

You may ask: 'what the heck is a frenemy'? Simply put, it is person who *says* they are your friend but *acts* like an enemy. It is your girlfriend who, when the chips are down and you need someone in your corner, is nowhere to be found (either physically or emotionally). It can be disheartening, disappointing, and depending on how embedded she is in your life…downright painful!

An example: You come into the room sashaying your 'new look', fresh from the salon, and your frenemy says "did you do something to your hair?" with a negative tone, straight face and squinted eyes. Quickly deflating any new sense of confidence you had just acquired through the magical hands of your stylist. Making you doubt your own taste and yourself. It is just how we women are built. We look to our friends for confirmation of our new looks and ourselves.

Another example: You call your frenemy enthusiastically, with great news and whole-heartedly expect her to join you in your joy. She proceeds to rain on your parade with questions and comments on all the reasons it cannot possibly work or there must be a "catch", it cannot possibly be that good, instead of enjoying the moment with you. All the while, saying she is just being "realistic" and does not want you to get your hopes up. Why not? Why not get your hopes up?! Through hope comes change! Hope is a wonderful healing emotion and can be a catalyst for change. Quickly excuse yourself from the conver-sation before your frenemy quickly and completely douses your dreams and enthusiasm.

I am sorry to say, but she was never a friend. You actually had a frenemy on the inside (inside your home, social circle, or heart). We, as women, look to each other for positive support and encourage-ment. A safe place.

When the people you surround yourself with are not lifting you up, it is time to cut your losses and move on. How do you know if you have a frenemy in your life? Here are some questions to ask yourself:

> How do you feel when you are with your friend? Do you feel uplifted and a general sense of well-being?
>
> Do you hear her saying small, unsupportive, passive-aggressive comments towards you?
>
> Do her actions match her words?
>
> Biggest indicator: your gut. Your intuition always knows even if you do not want to listen! Do a 'gut check' and see how you feel. Simply put: Do you feel better or worst after spending time with her? Best indicator of all! We always know even when we do not want too. Your intuition can be screaming at you and you are saying,' no, not Susie, she would never do that'. We have instincts for a reason; trust them.

Look around your circle of friends. You should see a wonderful group of people who you enjoy and trust and who ultimately, make your life better. If not, then it might be time to do some emotional de-cluttering. We, at Mama Bootcamp, call it the 'sister code'. Laugh with one another, cheer each other on, and support one another, knowing they will have your back, when the chips are down. Life can be challenging, you need your circle to be clean and healthy!

Friendships can be for a SEASON a REASON or a *Lifetime*

I love the quote above. Simple, right? Oprah says (and I paraphrase): "My best friend cheers for me the loudest when I am doing well, and is there for me with open arms when I fall".

ACTION PLAN NO. 27

Take a close look at your "circle." Does it include a frenemy? Or even more than one? If so, reevaluate her/his role in your life, and decide to make a change. Tell her/him what you think, and what you need. Or simply decide to elevate your circle to no longer include her/him in it.

Initially this might feel uncomfortable, and even scary. But ultimately, you will only be the better for it. When you are surrounded by true friends, the world is a much more supportive and happy place.

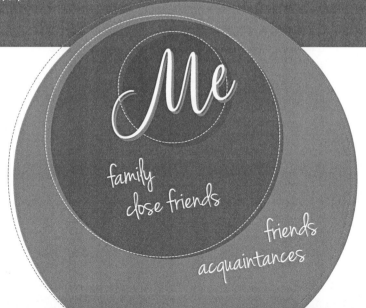

Me

family
close friends

friends
acquaintances

[CHALLENGE 28] FORGIVENESS

Writing this book has stirred up a lot of mixed emotions. I have had to look at my own participation in my life, whether it be conscious or otherwise. After all, I picked the players involved. I ignored red flags: a 'whisper' from intuition, loud blaring 'in my face' sorts of message to STOP....yet I continued, sometimes not trusting my inner voice trying to teach me the easy way. I used to look at the world with rose-colored glasses, thinking that people were never really deceitful... or selfish... or greedy... or downright mean. When I knew in my heart-of-hearts that there was something 'off', I often proceeded willingly and cheerfully down a dark alley with people I had no business trusting or being with! Why was I not trusting my inner voice screaming at me to *not* go!?

I did not trust myself, so the lessons kept coming at me in different bodies and jobs and living situations until I finally got *it*.

Where in your life are you having a gut reaction... an intuition about something but 'poo-poohing' it off by saying, "No, not her... or him or them"? Not trusting *you*... just like I did. Hard lessons had to be learned because I did not listen; some of them life-threatening. *Nothing* is worse than not being true to yourself.

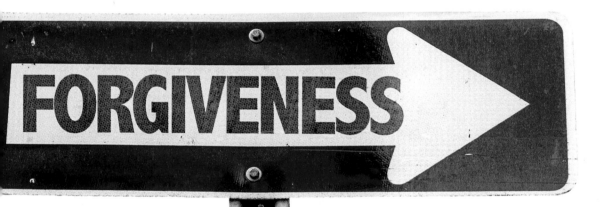

Think about situations where the theme has been the same, with different players. Do you keep picking the same sort of partner, friends, or job situations? Do you say "WHY does this ALWAYS happen to me?" Are you being lied to over and over? Is 'betrayal' a theme in your life? Are you continually putting yourself LAST on your list and being treated like a doormat by those you care about? Are you saying, "here I go again, different day, same situation?" Areas to look at: finances, living situations, job situations, self-destructive behaviors (including self-sabotage), friendships, family relationships.

Buy a journal and look for a similar theme and write them down. What is the lesson? Trust yourself to know. Just start writing and it will come to you.

When I started this chapter on "forgiveness", I was thinking of those that betrayed me, *not* of my bad choices. It just sort of evolved, this deep sense of shame in my life choices. The person I needed to forgive was *me*. Forgiving myself for bad choices, for accepting bad behavior from a boyfriend or girlfriend or business situation, as well as other self-destructive behaviors.

The bottom line: when you know better, you do better! There were lessons I needed to learn. The lesson will *keep* reappearing in different forms until you truly learn from it, and let it go. Painful yes; but definitely necessary.

[CHALLENGE 29] STEPPING THROUGH THE FEAR

In July of 1999, my husband was pounding on the door trying to get "back" in the house, after telling me in a drunken rage that he was leaving me (a repeat theme for the last year). Having three children 6 years old and younger, I was trying my best to keep calm and keep my husband from coming in. Full of fear and deciding to try and reason with him, I was frantically trying to unlock the door, but before I could get the deadbolt undone, he busted the door open and off the hinges. Turning to run, I swooped up my youngest child under my arm. Feeling a square thud on my back between my shoulder blades, I realized he had thrown his truck keys at me since I was out of the reach of his fists. I grabbed the phone, ran out the back door with my daughter under my arm and frantically called 911, screaming into the phone *"Get here now, my husband is going to kill me"*. Sober enough to realize I had just called the police, he stopped hitting my back as I covered my daughter with my body. He ran to his truck, peeling out of the driveway, and he was apprehended by the police in front of our house.

I was afraid, exhausted, and full of anxiety. I had no job, no family, was isolated and frightened about the future and I was paralyzed. Deer in the headlights; frozen and not able to move.

I know now that many people have been in situations where they are so overwhelmed with fear and other emotions that they stay afraid of the consequences of leaving. I have heard it said that "the devil you know, is better than the devil you don't". We stay in situations that slowly suck away our

You have to name it to claim it and feel it to heal it… not always pleasant but necessary.

Then forgive yourself for choosing the same people in different bodies, job situations, etc. Tell yourself (mirror work is especially effective here): "I am sorry that I treated you badly, accepting situations you do not deserve. Moving forward, I will try my best to honor you and treat you with the love you deserve."

Say this to yourself several times a day until it is absorbed into your body and soul. Write it and share it with someone you trust. You will be surprised at how much lighter you feel and how freeing it can be! The result will be new self-love, free of guilt of being in situations that did not support you.

Be kind to yourself in the process, because it is a process and may take a little while. Sending you blessings and light during this weekly challenging – you are worth getting to the other side.

ACTION PLAN NO. 28

ACTION PLAN NO. 29

Write down areas or situations you would like to no longer being paralyzed by. Get help from a friend or professional and come up with a game plan. Visit a college counselor if it is a new career. Talk to a family therapist if it is around your marriage and/or family.

Life coaches are fantastic for helping you with career and life situations. Even the internet is a plethora of information if you need free advice just to start exploring. Try to have fun with it! Set up an accountability buddy or schedule time with someone to practice asking for what you need. Take a chance, step through, you will not regret seeing courage in yourself that you did not know you had. Oh, and one last thought:

Being fearless is not having "no fear" It is *moving forward* in spite of being afraid.

hope, happiness, and life... Frozen and afraid to move in any direction because it might be the wrong direction or choice.

For me, what finally got me moving forward was the love for my children. Afraid my boys would grow up to be abusers and my daughter would think abuse is normal in relationships (after all, I said it was okay by staying). Eventually, I did it for myself. It took a while, as I was still working on self-love.

Here is what I know to be true: you cannot go under, around, or over fear. In order to minimize and eliminate fear, you must step through it. You are not living your life fully if you stay stuck in fear.

What situations are making you feel stuck, overwhelmed or afraid to move? Is your job unfulfilling and are you "living" only for your days off? Does applying for jobs or going back to school seem overwhelming so you just do nothing? Same with a bad relationship: does untangling finances and property keep you there? Afraid to be "alone", willing to put up with bad behavior because after all... who would want you?

These are real situations that I have had mamas share with me. Sometimes, training to do something you previously thought you could not, like learning to swim and competing in your first triathlon or first 5K fun run stretches your self-belief enough to know you *can* do it!

You are capable and have a wealth of resources and strength at your fingertips, inside of you, but you will never know until you try. Baby steps, my friend. One day at a time, one week. Layering on moments of success until you are on the other side!

[CHALLENGE 30] RANDOM ACTS OF KINDNESS

Being kind to others – notice the ripple effect back to you. Being kind is probably a part of your everyday life. After all, you have to be nice, in general, to get what you want and to keep the people you love happy.

But what about being kind simply for the sake of being kind? What about doing something kind for someone you don't need anything from, or even someone you don't know?

Practicing kindness, and passing it on to others encourages others to do the same thing. If we are all being kind, and doing kind things for each other, the world is bound to be a better place. And doing something nice for someone "just because" creates a feel- good moment for the giver and recipient!

I believe kindness is undervalued and underrated. Kind people are generally looked at as weak and easy to take advantage of. I personally feel there is great compassion and strength in kindness. It takes courage to stick up for someone who is being bullied for whatever reason. When you are having a rough day or week, being kind to someone *else* can actually make *you* feel better! Plus, whatever you give out comes back to you ten-fold and creates great karma at the same time: win/win.

When I was going through a particularly bad year (wishing it was only going to be a month at the most), I literally would envelope myself in kindness, seeking out situations where I could give a little something back, knowing I would feel some sort of relief. One day, after feeling especially despondent, I stood next to a group of volunteers at an event and let their good 'juju' wash over me as they were laughing, lifting the veil of depression off of me for a few minutes. I remember feeling some moments of relief.

Words, actions, sounds can be full of kindness. The vibrations of the laughter and uplifting words were contagious and truly powerful.

Make it a point to go out of your way to bring a smile to someone's face to lift their spirits. It can be something as small as wishing a person to *"have a great day"*. That alone might be words someone holds onto... I know it was for me.

ACTION PLAN NO. 30

Do something kind for someone at least once daily! Offer kind words to a stranger, offer a helping hand to someone who needs it, pay for someone's coffee (remember when that went on at the local Starbucks?), mow someone's lawn, move someone's trash can in on garbage day, leave a kind note on someone's door. Leave a complimentary note for a co-worker, family member, friend. Send someone a letter of appreciation. Send an email of thanks. Send flowers. Purchase and leave a bag of groceries for a struggling student or family or senior. Tell your boss or employee how much you appreciate them.

NEED SOME MORE GREAT IDEAS? VISIT THE RANDOM ACTS OF KINDNESS FOUNDATION AT WWW.RANDOMACTSOFKINDNESS.ORG

JULY IN REVIEW

FOR JULY
MY GOALS

FOR JULY
MY GRATITUDE LIST

FOR JULY
RELATIONSHIPS TO INVEST IN

FOR JULY
WHAT'S GOING WELL

FOR JULY
WHAT NEEDS TO CHANGE

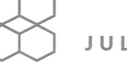

JULY NOTES

(lined note paper)

MY DOODLE SQUARE

AUGUST

FITNESS: YOUR BODY EITHER SERVES YOU, OR LIMITS YOU

IT IS AMAZING TO ME AT HOW RESILIENT THE BODY CAN BE. HOW BADLY WE CAN TREAT IT AND WHEN WE CHANGE OUR MINDS, DECIDE TO MAKE BETTER CHOICES AROUND FOOD AND MOVEMENT, JUST HOW QUICKLY THE BODY CAN RESPOND IN A POSITIVE AND RESTORATIVE WAY. IT IS AS IF THE BODY IS JUST WAITING FOR YOU TO PLEASE, PLEASE TAKE CARE OF ME!

I REMEMBER A WOMAN NAMED KATE, WHOM I STARTED WORKING WITH WHEN I WAS PERSONAL TRAINING AT A LOCAL RACQUET CLUB. KATE CAME TO ME TELLING ME SHE HAD TO MAKE A CHANGE OR DIE. SHE WAS LITERALLY DRINKING HERSELF TO DEATH. SHE HAD SEEN THE CHAOS OF DRUG AND ALCOHOL ADDICTION IN HER IMMEDIATE FAMILY'S LIFE AND WAS FOLLOWING DOWN THAT SAME PATH. SHE WAS FEARFUL - JUST COMING FROM THE DOCTOR'S OFFICE, HEARING HER LIVER ENZYMES WERE UP AND THAT SHE NEEDED TO MAKE CHANGES IMMEDIATELY.

AFTER YEARS OF DRINKING AND SEEING THE DAMAGING EFFECTS, SHE DECIDED TO QUIT AND TRULY COMMIT TO THE PROCESS. IT WAS AMAZING HOW QUICKLY HER BODY RESPONDED. DRINKING LOTS OF WATER, EATING FRESH FRUITS AND VEGGIES, AND GIVING UP ALCOHOL HELPED WITH HER TRAINING AND HER LIFE. NEXT, SHE DECIDED TO TRAIN FOR A RACE, HER FIRST 5K (3 MILE FUN RUN) AND WANTED TO RUN THE WHOLE THING, NO WALKING! FAST FORWARD TO NOW, KATE IS ALCOHOL FREE, A RUNNER AND TRIATHLETE, AND TRULY LOVING LIFE! THE BODY ALWAYS SAYS "YES" TO HEALTH!

IT IS NEVER TOO LATE TO "CHANGE YOUR MIND" AND START TREATING YOUR BODY WITH THE LOVE AND CARE IT DESERVES. TAKE CARE OF YOUR BODY SO IT CAN TAKE CARE OF YOU!

[CHALLENGE 31] WEEKLY BODY CARE

One year I trained very very hard with minimal rest or days off, plus life got crazy busy! I felt I had no "extra" time for body care! This meant no stretching, no foam rolling, no "nothing"! I kept pushing and training for races and all the while multi-tasking the heck out of every hour while Mama Bootcamp kept expanding and growing. Finally, my body said *"no more!"*, stopping me dead in my tracks. Yelling at me to listen! Back pain, knee issues, plantar fasciitis, and micro tears in my achilles tendon all made me STOP and take heed! This brought all my racing and training to a screeching halt. I was forced to stop so my body could take some much needed healing time and catch up on recovery. *Not* fun when it is your joy and your business. Listening to my own advice, I took some well-deserved rest and recovered, spending time in physical therapy and with the techniques listed below.

I am encouraging, nudging, pushing you to heed my advice with this chapter and listen first to your body and then to me.

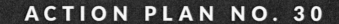

ACTION PLAN NO. 30

Try, and then put into practice, one of these weekly body care techniques. I suggest rotating so each is done at least once over the course of the month. The benefits are HUGE and all of the above are designed to have wonderful side effects of injury free training, flushing toxins, and keeping your body a fine tuned and well-oiled machine to keep you moving. At a minimum, it will speed up recovery and keep your training fluid and smooth. Maximally, it will prevent injury and possibly surgery! So do not wait until your body screeches to a halt… schedule your weekly "ahhhhh" on your calendar.

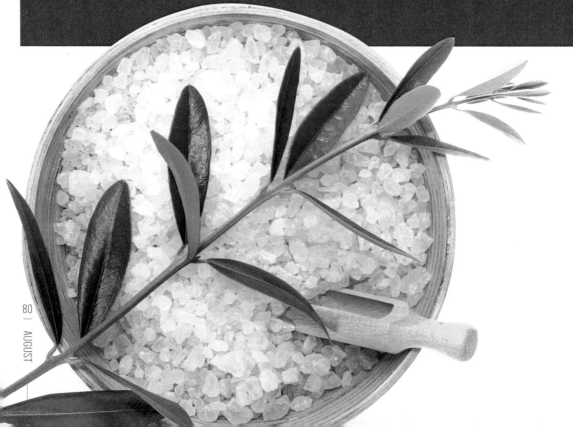

FOAM ROLLING

Using a foam roller to "work out the kinks" is a quick and easy way to release sore spots, tight IT band and glut muscles. It is also great for hips, calves, back, quads, and lats. If a connective tissue like a tendon is tight, it can yank on your knees, low back, shoulders, neck, etc. and create a larger issue if not corrected. Pick one up on Amazon.com, (they often have the best prices). The right "roll" for the job can keep you moving and injury free!

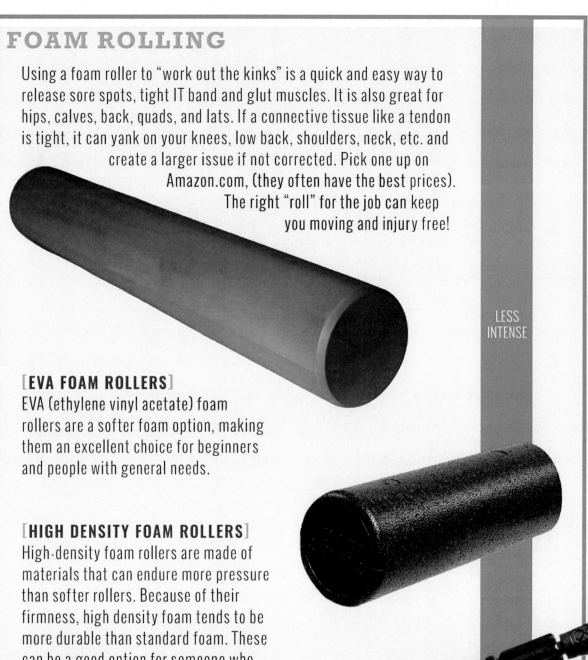

LESS INTENSE

[EVA FOAM ROLLERS]
EVA (ethylene vinyl acetate) foam rollers are a softer foam option, making them an excellent choice for beginners and people with general needs.

[HIGH DENSITY FOAM ROLLERS]
High-density foam rollers are made of materials that can endure more pressure than softer rollers. Because of their firmness, high density foam tends to be more durable than standard foam. These can be a good option for someone who prefers a deeper massage.

[TEXTURED OR RIBBED ROLLERS]
These are firm foam rollers that are covered with bumps or ridges that provide a little extra massage. These rollers contain a solid core that help maintain their durability and allowing for a deeper, high-pressure feel.

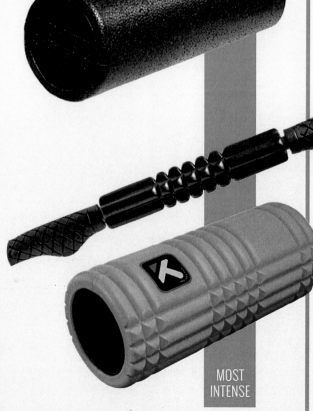

MOST INTENSE

ICE MASSAGE

Fill a small paper cup (hot foam cups work best) with water and freeze. When frozen, peel the top down about a quarter to half inch. Use this to massage in a circular movement on areas that are tight or sore. The ice acts as an anti-inflammatory to help ease pain and inflammation that can come after a hard workout. I especially like this on my shins after a plyometric workout or long run on uneven terrain (like a trail run). Studies show that icing muscles is one of the best ways to recover without contra indications from a workout and furthermore can reduce the risk of injury! A great way to stop plantar fasciitis is to freeze a 16.9 ounce water bottle and roll your foot over it for 5 minutes at a time, breaking up the tight tendon at the bottom of the foot and releasing knots.

MASSAGE / PHYSICAL THERAPY

Self massage, your partner, or professional massage are all amazing ways to recover! Massage manipulates a faster recovery by moving muscle waste by-products, toxins, and lactic acid out of the muscle tissue. And who doesn't love a great massage? Physical therapy as prevention is also a wonderful tool especially if you are training for longer events (anything half marathon or longer is my recommendation). Find a great sports physical therapist by asking friends for recommendations.

EPSOM SALT SOAK

Add two cups into a hot bath and soak for 15 to 20 minutes. It will help draw out toxins and an added bonus… you will sleep like a baby! Bonus bonus: super soft skin! After draining your bath, rinse off your body with a quick shower or large cups of water to rinse the toxins off that were just drawn out. Remember to hydrate as this does have a tendency to dehydrate you because of the "drawing" properties! If you have any type of blood sugar issues, please consult your doctor. Type 1 or Type II diabetics are not advised for salt baths so please consult your physician.

THE ICE PLUNGE

I like to say if an "ice plunge" is good enough for multi-millionaire athletes, it is certainly good enough for my mamas! Huge stainless steel vats of ice water await professional athletes after tough work outs and/or games so they can recover as quickly as possible. The "plunge" SNAPS everything (blood vessels and capillaries) shut! Forcing out the gunk (toxins) and pulling in blood flow (nutrients). If these highly paid athletes are using this as a recovery tool and anti-injury technique... why wouldn't we?

I like this after long workouts or plyometrics (like H.I.I.T. training). Think of it like this: you trained hard creating small micro tears in your muscles fibers. Your body wants to "pool" blood around these mini injuries that happen when you exercise. Eventually you heal and rebuild a stronger, tighter, firmer muscle. In the meantime (between the work and the heal), the stagnant pool around each muscle keeps you from recovering quickly so icing releases the inflammation so blood flow (bringing nutrients) can get to the suspected injury quicker, then healing the tear so you can get back to business quicker. Definitely an acquired taste, but oh so effective!

[**WHERE**] Use an unheated pool in your community or backyard, lake or river, or your own bathtub.

[**HOW**] Waist down is the best area to submerge: your legs and including your lower back in the process. I have been known to wear a warm jacket, sip hot tea, and read a good article on my phone (which is in a waterproof baggie), since recommended timing is 12 to 15 minutes. You want to get the blood flow cold and below the surface of the skin and into the deep tissue, since this is bringing the cool blood to the tissue that needs healing. Please allow the body to warm up slowly because this is where the healing happens on its own (no jumping into a hot tub right after... the "slow warming" is necessary). It is such a great and effective technique, **but** definitely an acquired taste.

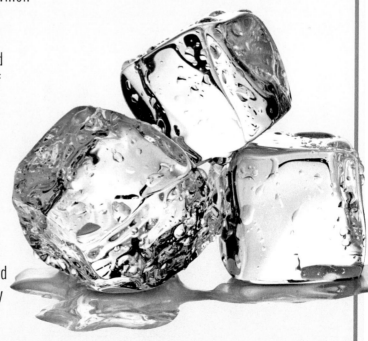

BODY CARE 101

[CHALLENGE 32] BACK ATTACK

Back problems… yikes!!! Nothing affects your quality of life faster than back problems. You cannot move easily and without pain and certainly you cannot exercise. Afraid of moving for fear it will make it worse, you stop and everything gets tighter, triggering even more issues. You cannot sleep well so your healing capacity (yes… you heal when you sleep) is at a huge disadvantage. My goal with this challenge is for you to incorporate the Back Attack into your daily routine. It takes only five minutes and literally can be life changing. The series of four movements are yoga and Pilates-based, and they strengthen and stretch the muscles on either side of the spine. They purposefully alternate between the two exercise types.

ACTION PLAN NO. 32

Perform the Back Attack daily at the same time of the day so it becomes a health habit and part of your lifestyle. This takes five minutes maximum, doing each pose in succession 10 times each. Your back will say "**thank you**" and remain strong, flexible, healthy, and happy so you can move through the world pain free.

BACK ATTACK!

DAILY AT THE SAME TIME OF THE DAY. TOTAL OF FIVE MINUTES MAXIMUM, DOING EACH POSE IN SUCCESSION 10 TIMES EACH.

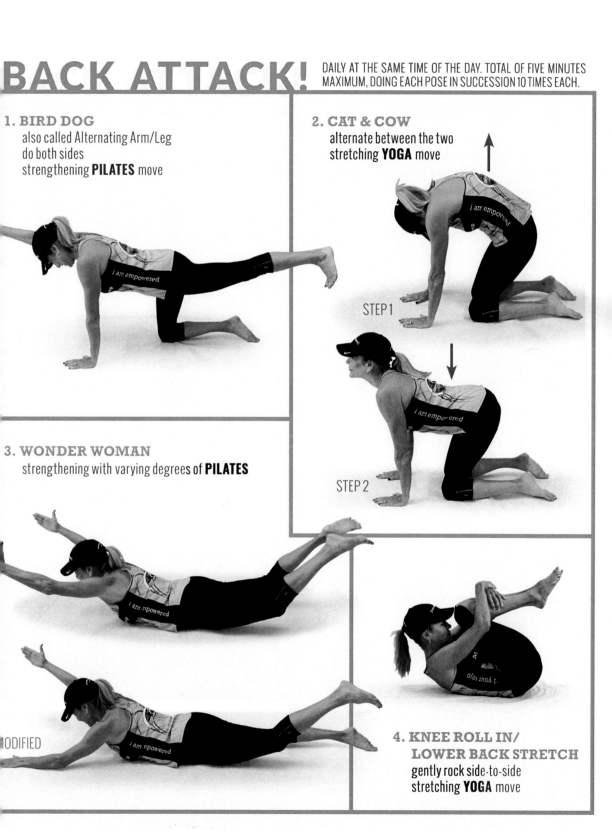

1. BIRD DOG
also called Alternating Arm/Leg
do both sides
strengthening **PILATES** move

2. CAT & COW
alternate between the two
stretching **YOGA** move

STEP 1

STEP 2

3. WONDER WOMAN
strengthening with varying degrees of **PILATES**

MODIFIED

4. KNEE ROLL IN/ LOWER BACK STRETCH
gently rock side-to-side
stretching **YOGA** move

[CHALLENGE 33] THE F.I.T.T. PRINCIPLE

THE F.I.T.T. PRINCIPLE IS A WAY TO CROSS TRAIN USING THE SAME MODALITY SUCH AS RUNNING, WALKING, CYCLING, SWIMMING, ETC. YOU CAN EVEN USE THIS IN YOUR OWN LOCAL GYM OR DURING STRENGTH TRAINING!

I get bored easily and often say I have "attention deficit disorder" when it comes to exercise. Now I know this is actually a good thing for results, albeit challenging because of the creativity factor! We need to constantly mix it up to avoid boredom and in addition... the adaptation process. The adaption process is your body getting used to doing the same thing when repeated. The better shape you are in, the quicker you adapt to the "load" (workout). So changing your work out every four to six weeks maximum is very important if you want to keep getting "results" (weight loss, muscle development, faster speeds).

1. **F**REQUENCY
2. **I**NTENSITY
3. **T**IME
4. **T**YPE

I am sure you have heard of "hitting a plateau". Usually this term is reserved for weight loss. You have been doing the same thing over and over and your body has adapted and you are stuck. In order to keep moving forward (whether it is for losing weight or enhancing endurance), you need to surprise the body! You see it all the time in infomercials... "shock the body"! So now you know the secret, and you can do this on your own by following the F.I.T.T. Principle.

To monitor the "Intensity" of the F.I.T.T. Principle, you can use your "Rate of Perceived Exertion", or R.P.E. Basically R.P.E. means "how are you feeling?" on a scale from 1 to 10, with 1 being completely still and 10 being an all-out sprint. You can modulate the intensity of your runs (or any workout) by adding speed, hills, more weight, more reps, or more time. This is a wonderful way to have fun while moving!

RATE OF PERCEIVED EXERTION

10 — **MAX EFFORT**
YOU'RE UNABLE TO TALK

9 — **EXTREMELY VIGOROUS ACTIVITY**
YOU'RE VERY SHORT OF BREATH

7-8 — **VIGOROUS ACTIVITY**
YOU'RE SHORT OF BREATH

4-6 — **MODERATE ACTIVITY**
YOU'RE BREATHING HEAVILY

2-3 — **LIGHT ACTIVITY**
YOU CAN BREATH AND CONVERSE

1 — **VERY LIGHT ACTIVITY**
YOU'RE AT REST

SAMPLE F.I.T.T. PRINCIPLE WORKOUT WEEK

Say you are running 30 minutes per day Monday through Friday on the same route near your home after work. Saturday and Sunday are your rest days. You are bored, and you are noticing it has gotten pretty easy. You are looking less forward to your daily run. Using the F.I.T.T. Principle, you decide to mix it up. Your "type" of workout stays the same: type = running. However, you mix up your running schedule by modifying the three other parts of the F.I.T.T. Principle: "Frequency", "Intensity" and "Time".

SUNDAY	Start by adding five minutes to your run time. Work up to adding 90 minutes of running time. (Remember the ten percent rule: do not add any more than ten percent weekly to avoid injury).
MONDAY	keep the same as Sunday.
TUESDAY	you know you can get on the track at the local high school and add stadium laps, doing a 4 lap warmup. Work your way up to 10 laps.
WEDNESDAY	an easy run for 20 minutes, adding five minutes of core work beforehand.
THURSDAY	a 30 minute run on the local trail before work. You may find that you love seeing the sun come up on a trail run.
FRIDAY	Rest Day
SATURDAY	Rest Day

So you went from Monday through Friday of BLAH! to a fun mix of workouts; varying distances, places, tempos, and times to incorporate cross-training into your running!

ACTION PLAN NO. 33

Use at least two of the F.I.T.T. principles to mix up your workouts. If you want to get really crazy, use all four and plan on mixing it up again in four weeks. Have a friend, personal trainer, or coach hold you accountable. See the results roll in and the boredom roll out!

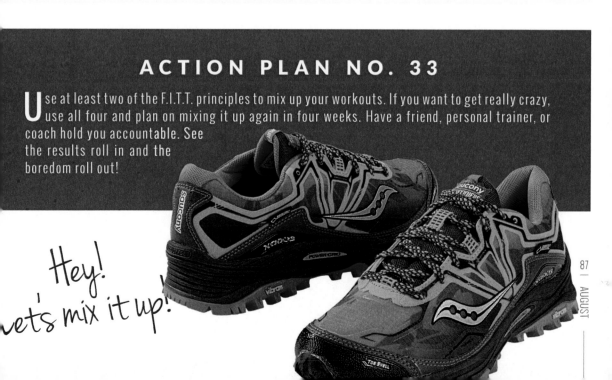

Hey! let's mix it up!

[CHALLENGE 34] GET YOUR ZZZZZ'S

The power of sleep... restorative and rejuvenating, it is a cornerstone to finding your mojo. When I do not get enough sleep, I feel lethargic, exhausted, and downright depressed. It is hard for me to find energy and zest for life when I am dragging throughout my day. In addition, burning the candle at both ends burns me out and makes me less productive. Sleep is *soooo* important and needs to be a priority! I actually schedule time to sleep in at least once a week.

A great example is one of our Mamas, Sue. Sue was having a very challenging time with insomnia. Unable to think clearly or problem solve was affecting every area of her life. Irritable and exhausted, sleepless nights were taking their toll on her job, marriage, and career. She had even tried prescription medications, but did not like the after-effects upon waking.

By the time we met for her intake to get started with Mama Bootcamp, she was desperate for help and willing to jump in with both feet. Sue committed to three days a week of Bootcamp, plus two days of walking for 30 minutes during her lunch. Noticing her mood improve and generally feeling better after the first week, she was hopeful. After one month of consistency, she actually started sleeping through the night and felt more energized throughout her day! In the process, she dropped 25 pounds and starting training for triathlons and half marathons... talk about finding your mojo!

REASONS TO MAKE SURE YOU ARE MAKING TIME TO HIT THE PILLOW

✓ Lack of sleep causes accidents. Drowsiness can slow reaction time as much as driving drunk.

✓ Sleep plays a critical role in thinking and learning. Lack of sleep hurts these cognitive processes. It impairs attention, alertness, concentration, reasoning, and problem solving. This makes it more difficult to learn efficiently.

✓ Sleep deprivation and chronic sleep loss can lead to serious health problems and put you at risk for heart disease, irregular heartbeat, high blood pressure, stroke, and diabetes.

✓ Insomnia is often one of the first symptoms of depression. Sleep loss often aggravates the symptoms of depression, and depression can make it more difficult to fall asleep.

✓ Lack of sleep ages you. When you don't get enough sleep, your body releases more of the stress hormone cortisol. In excess amounts, cortisol can break down skin collagen, the protein that keeps skin smooth and elastic. Sleep loss also causes the body to release too little human growth hormone. As we age, it helps increase muscle mass, thicken skin, and strengthen bones.

✓ Losing sleep can promote gain weight. Lack of sleep seems to be related to an increase in hunger and appetite, and possibly to obesity. Not only does sleep loss appear to stimulate appetite, it also stimulates cravings for high-fat, high-carbohydrate foods. People who sleep less than six hours a day were almost thirty percent more likely to become obese than those who slept seven to nine hours.

✓ Sleep is when your body heals and recovers. Body builders, an extreme population, but one we can learn from, actually take sleep aides so they can sleep longer for maximum recovery from grueling workouts and grow more lean muscle tissue. When you start an exercise program, you may notice your need for sleep increases. Your body needs more time in rest to gain the benefits from your workouts!

ACTION PLAN NO. 34

TIPS TO GETTING A WONDERFUL NIGHT OF ZZZZZ'S

Cut the caffeine. Coffee in the morning is fine, but as soon as the clock strikes noon, avoid caffeine in foods and drinks. Caffeine interferes with the deeper stages of sleep.

Rethink drinking alcohol at bedtime. Alcohol actually disrupts the deep REM sleep making your less likely to get a great nights rest.

Turn off TVs, computers, and other blue light producers an hour before sleep. Cover any blue displays you can't shut off. The short waves of blue light may interfere with sleep.

Use caution when taking sleeping pills. Some sleep medicines can be habit forming and may have bothersome side effects. Ideally, they should be used as a very short-term solution, while other lifestyle and behavior changes are put in place.

Set your body clock. Go to sleep and wake up at about the same time every day —including weekends. This routine will put your brain and body on a healthy sleep-wake cycle. In time, you'll be able to fall asleep quickly and sleep soundly through the night. Get out in bright light for 5 to 30 minutes as soon as you rise. Light is the most powerful regulator of the biological clock.

Lower the lights and neutralize noise. Starting two to three hours before bedtime, dim the lights around the house and put aside any work. It takes time to turn off the emotional and intellectual "noise" of the day. Lowering the lights signals your brain to produce melatonin, the hormone that brings on sleep.

Soothing "white noise" covers up bumps in the night. You can use a fan, an air-conditioner, or a white noise generator available in stores. Ear plugs also work.

Eat right at night. Avoid heavy foods and big meals late in the day; they tax the digestive system and make it hard to get high-quality sleep.

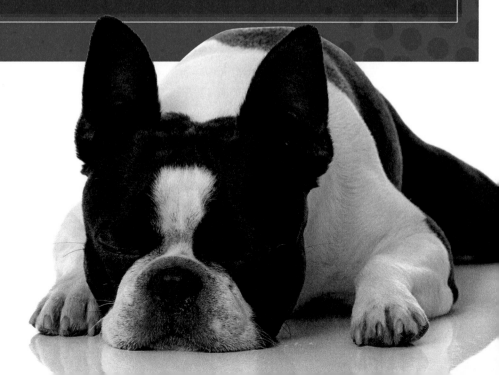

AUGUST IN REVIEW

MY GOALS

MY GRATITUDE LIST

RELATIONSHIPS TO INVEST IN

WHAT'S GOING WELL

WHAT NEEDS TO CHANGE

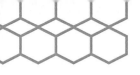

AUGUST NOTES

_____
_____
_____
_____
_____
_____
_____
_____
_____
_____
_____
_____
_____
_____
_____
_____
_____
_____
_____
_____
_____
_____
_____
_____
_____
_____
_____

MY DOODLE SQUARE

SEPTEMBER

NUTRITION: BAM!

IN FINDING YOUR MOJO, THE MOST IMPORTANT PIECE...OR AT LEAST EQUALLY IMPORTANT TO MOVEMENT, IS FOOD! WE ARE RUNNING AROUND AT A FASTER PACE THAN EVER AND OFTEN FIND OURSELVES IN FAST FOOD LINES STARVING! AND AFTERWARDS, QUICKLY REMEMBER WHY WE NEVER WANT TO DO THAT AGAIN. FEELING LADEN WITH FAT, SALT, AND CALORIES, WE PROMISE OURSELVES TO PREPARE BETTER AND PACK SNACKS. AND YET, INEVITABLY, IT HAPPENS AGAIN. POOR PLANNING, CRAZY SCHEDULES, AND SQUISHED FOR TIME, THERE WE ARE AGAIN IN LINE....WAITING TO RE-LOAD. WONDERING HOW THIS COULD HAPPEN YET AGAIN. THIS MONTH IS ALL ABOUT TREATING YOUR BODY LIKE YOU WANT IT TO TREAT YOU. PREPPING FOR YOUR WEEK, TRYING SOME NEW THINGS TO GET OUT OF A NUTRITIONAL RUT, AND MAKING SURE YOU ARE GETTING ENOUGH PROTEIN TO RE-BUILD BEAUTIFUL LEAN MUSCLE! PLUS, KEEPING IT SIMPLE SO IT WORKS FOR YOU. CLEAN AND HEALTHY EATING HERE YOU COME...NUTRITIONAL BAM!

ACTION PLAN NO. 35

Saturday is shopping day! You shop for fresh fruits, veggies, lean protein, etc. Prepare your menu and grocery list, focusing on keeping it simple.

Sunday is your prep day (or pick another day of the week that works for you; just keep it consistent). Wash and chop your veggies and other meals by 6:00 p.m. Prepare as much of your food as you can for the week (yogurt parfaits for breakfasts, Mojo in a Jar salads, etc.)

With minimal pre-preparing and preplanning, you will be feeling fantastic and ready to take on the world... imagine that!

[CHALLENGE 35] FEED YOUR BODY THE GOOD STUFF

We all have a tendency to get stuck in nutritional ruts... always eating the same thing when we are trying to eat "clean". On the flip side, when we start to eat crap and therefore feel like "crap" it is hard to pull ourselves up by the boot straps and get back on the right path. It is like the more I eat fast food, sugar, salt, etc. the *more* I want! Who has woken up on a Monday with cotton brain and puffy eyes from sugar/salt/alcohol overload? I know I have, and it generally takes two days to recover from a few days away from your game plan.

This month is about getting on track and staying there by keeping it interesting, fun, flavorful, and creative and clean. Pack your lunch and take it to work every day! Choose whole grains, fresh fruits and veggies, and zero foods with no strange words you cannot pronounce. No eating out! Think of the money you will save! You can even put that money in a jar to motivate you to stay on track.

Here is what has been my solution and also can be yours. Sunday night has become my prep night for the week. If I spend a couple hours Sunday night getting

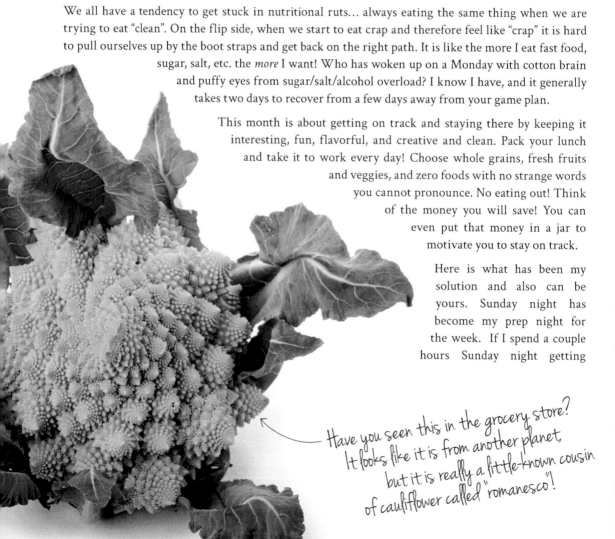

Have you seen this in the grocery store? It looks like it is from another planet, but it is really a little-known cousin of cauliflower called "romanesco"!

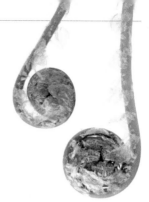

ready for the week, it's pretty much a given that I will eat clean, healthy meals the rest of the week. There are so many things you can make quickly that will help make sure your meals are ready fast! If you spend a couple hours Sunday night, you can get breakfast for the week made, lunch prepared, have fresh fruit and vegetables ready to snack on or for smoothies, and have pasta or grilled chicken and vegetables ready to add to any meal!

[CHALLENGE 36] TRY SOMETHING NEW!

Am I eating the same things on the same days week after week? Fall is around the corner and it feels like Groundhog Day. Nothing feels new or fresh. Am I alone? Or do some of you feel the same way too? This week's challenge is about breaking out of the rut, monotony, doldrums or whatever you want to call it...Trying something new might lead to a wonderful new "favorite" food or recipe.

While at your local grocery store or farmer's market, look for produce that is unfamiliar to you. Ask the grocer what it is and how to prepare it. Browse a local bookstore (or look online) for interesting cookbooks or articles. One of my favorites is *Vegetables: Made Easy with Step-by-Step Photographs,* from Williams Sonoma (see details in Resources on page 131). In this book, different "types" of vegetables are explained (leafy greens, brassicas, roots, tubers, pods & seeds, vegetable fruits, squashes, stalks and alliums) and the best techniques to use for preparing, cooking and serving.

ACTION PLAN NO. 35

Find one new recipe to try this month. Find two new varieties of fruit or vegetable to try this month. Explore your unknown, mix it up and have fun!

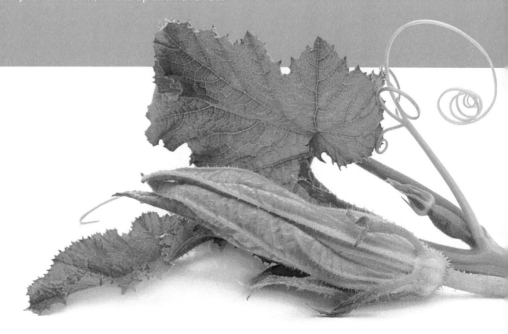

[CHALLENGE 37]
RECOVER FROM YOUR WORKOUT WITH PROTEIN

With the overwhelming variety of sports foods available today, it can be difficult to figure out what to eat to fuel your workouts. Before gels, bars, or sports drinks, it is important to note that the best way that you can prepare your body for a workout is to properly recover from your previous workout.

Your recovery foods should include protein for muscle recovery, along with glycogen-replenishing carbohydrates.

THE BENEFITS OF PROTEIN

✓ BUILDS LEAN MUSCLE TISSUE AND AIDS IN MUSCLE RECOVERY AFTER WORKOUTS.

✓ HELPS TO KEEP BLOOD SUGAR EVEN TO AVOID "BONKING" DURING EXERCISE.

✓ PREVENTS CARB AND SUGAR CRAVINGS AND MOOD SWINGS THAT COME WITH FLUCTUATING BLOOD SUGAR LEVELS.

✓ WORKS WITH CARBOHYDRATES TO REPLENISH YOUR GLYCOGEN STORES AFTER LONG WORKOUTS, HELPING TO PREPARE YOUR BODY FOR YOUR NEXT WORKOUT.

✓ GIVES YOUR MEALS STAYING POWER BY HELPING YOU TO FEEL FULL LONGER.

How should I refuel after a workout? Most dietitians recommend consuming a post-workout snack or meal that contains a moderate amount of protein (10-20 grams) within 30 minutes.

ACTION PLAN NO. 37
Fuel up (or refuel) with a protein shake. Your body will love you for it!

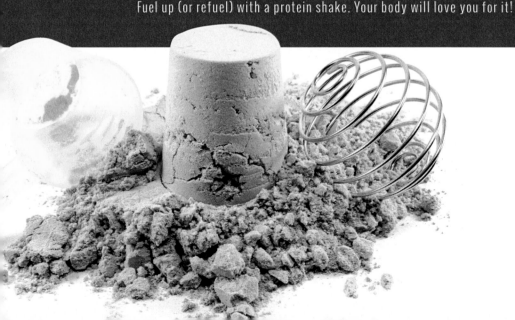

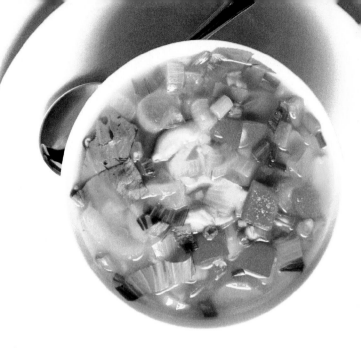

[CHALLENGE 38]
EAT YOUR
(VEGGIE) SOUP

In the winter, at least for me, it gets
a little harder to get in all seven to
nine servings of vegetables that my
body needs. When it is cold and rainy
outside, and all I want is comfort food,
a salad or crunchy carrots just doesn't
seem to fit the bill. That's where this
soup comes in. Warm and delicious, and
versatile enough to enjoy as a snack or a
full meal, veggie soup is comfort good that it
good for your body.

You can add whatever vegetables you like to this
soup. To change it up use a can of Rotel tomatoes
with mild green chilies, or add kidney beans, black, beans,
garbanzo beans, pinto beans or potatoes. You can also add turkey or chicken for a change.

ACTION PLAN NO. 38

Cook up a big pot of veggie soup on the first day of the challenge. Add your favorite veggies, or add some protein to make it a complete meal. Eat it when you need a snack, or a meal, or just something warm and delicious. Enjoy your comfort food, and know that you are doing something great for your body and your health.

3 tablespoons of **olive oil**
1 to 2 cloves of **fresh garlic**, diced
1 **onion**, chopped
3 to 4 **carrots**
3 to 4 (or more) 14 ounce cans of
chicken or vegetable broth
1 head of **cabbage**, chopped
3 to 4 **celery stalks**, chopped
1 **red bell pepper**, chopped
1 to 2 **yellow squash**, chopped
1 to 2 **green squash**, chopped
1 14 ounce can of **diced tomatoes**
½ teaspoon freshly ground **black pepper**
¼ cup chopped **fresh parsley leaves**
1 to 2 teaspoons **fresh lemon juice**

Heat the olive oil in a stockpot over medium-low heat. Once hot, add the onion, garlic and carrots, and brown until they begin to soften, approximately 7 to 8 minutes.

Add the broth, increase the heat to high, and bring to a simmer. Once simmering, add the cabbage, celery, bell pepper, squash, tomatoes and pepper. Reduce the heat to low, cover, and cook until the vegetables are fork tender, approximately 25 to 30 minutes. Remove from heat and add the parsley and lemon juice. Season, to taste, with kosher salt. Serve immediately.

MAKES 4 TO 6 SERVINGS

MAMA'S VEGGIE SOUP

SEPTEMBER IN REVIEW

FOR SEPTEMBER
MY GOALS

FOR SEPTEMBER
MY GRATITUDE LIST

FOR SEPTEMBER
RELATIONSHIPS TO INVEST IN

FOR SEPTEMBER
WHAT'S GOING WELL

FOR SEPTEMBER
WHAT NEEDS TO CHANGE

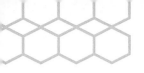

SEPTEMBER NOTES

_____
_____
_____
_____
_____
_____
_____
_____
_____
_____
_____
_____
_____
_____
_____
_____
_____
_____
_____
_____
_____
_____
_____
_____
_____
_____
_____

MY DOODLE SQUARE

OCTOBER

LIFE COACHING:
DON'T "FALL" OFF YOUR WAGON

FALL IS HERE. HARD TO BELIEVE, BUT THERE ARE ONLY THREE MONTHS LEFT IN THIS YEAR! YOU HAVE MADE GREAT PROGRESS WITH YOUR WEEKLY CHALLENGES AND ARE ALREADY REAPING THE REWARDS. LET'S STAY FOCUSED AS WE ENTER THE HOLIDAY SEASON AND NOT FALL OFF YOUR HARD-EARNED HABITS (WAGON) THAT YOU HAVE IMPLEMENTED.

[CHALLENGE 39] SEASONAL DISORDER

The weather is changing…dreary, foggy, and downright cold. The days are shorter without as much light, let alone sun shine. Your body wants to go into hibernation along with your brain. In addition, pressures of the holidays are coming with all the expectations of spending time with relatives you may not ever see except at the Thanksgiving and Christmas.

In addition, the added stretch on your finances with gift giving at home, the office, and other groups you may be involved. Sounds like a recipe for the blues! Personally, I am definitely affected by the change in seasons. I get bluesy, irritable, and down if left on my own. In order stay on track emotionally and mentally, I developed a bag of tricks to stay buoyant.

My bag of tricks involves things, people and places that bring me joy and lift my spirits. My "bag" includes going for a run, going to the movies, getting a pedicure or massage, going to bed early (a good night's sleep cures a lot for me), spending time with any one of my kids, playing with my dog Quincee, going to dinner with my hubby, talking to a one or two girlfriends who I can completely be myself with, donating time to those less fortunate, making a gratitude list, or planning a getaway. This is a partial list.

Some additional items on your list may be going to the mountains or ocean, reading a good book, doing an art project like painting or sculpting, getting a makeover at a local department store, going for a bike ride, walk on a local nature trail, spend time with anyone you totally trust or write in your journal.

Studies also show a wonderful relief for seasonal disorder is physical activity for 30 minutes or more per day. Endorphins are released! These chemicals are very real and tangible and will actually lift your mood!

ACTION PLAN NO. 35

Create your own "Bag of Tricks". Make a list of five "go-to's" when you feel the pressure of the season weighing on you. Brainstorm on ideas that have helped you in the past. Is there a particular place where you always feel warm and fuzzy? Who always lifts your spirit when you are with them? What activity brings you joy? Write them down and keep it in your wallet once completed. When you begin to feel the blues, pull out your list and get back on track to the path of positivity!

[CHALLENGE 40]
YOU HAVE THE RIGHT TO CHANGE YOUR MIND

One of our Mamas, Jane, shares her story to illustrate this point...

In my twenties, I was engaged to a young man who was attending college in my hometown. After college, he asked me to move home with him, five hours to the south. In retrospect, there were lots of red flags that I chose to ignore. However, I proceeded to plan to go anyway, thinking he was "the one".

The night before I was supposed to drive down with all of earthly belongings in a moving van, I had an overwhelming feeling that I should not go. I was sitting there with my best friend, Sandy, drinking a glass of champagne (after all, I was supposed to be celebrating, right?!) with a horrible sinking feeling in my gut.

I said to Sandy, "I don't want to go. I don't know why, but I just don't want to go."

And then she liberated me with two simple words... "Then don't". It was like someone threw a bucket of ice water on me and woke me up! I asked her, "Really? I don't have to go?"

Next I proceeded to list all the things I had done to get ready for my move.

"But I sold my car! What will I drive?" Sandy's reply: "You will just get another one."

"I already turned in my two weeks' notice for my job!" Sandy countered: "You will go to your boss and tell her you are staying, and she may give you your job back. But even if she doesn't, you will just get another job. I know you, and you will have no problem getting another one."

"I LOVE this place where I am living, but I offered it to a friend and she wants to rent it! What about that?" Sandy said: "Your friend will either understand, or not, but in the meantime, you have not moved out yet."

I looked at Sandy with relief and said, "Do you mean I really do not have to go?" And she said these magical words: **"You have the right to change your mind."** I was so unbelievably grateful for her faith in me. I was hearing a truth that I had never been taught: to honor my intuition and gut instinct, especially when it is yelling at me!

ACTION PLAN NO. 40

Think back to times when you listened to your intuition and it totally served you. Write it down in your journal for "proof" when you need it that your intuition is very real and to be trusted. You can trust you! Also make notes to when you did not listen and what the consequences were. Again just for research.

Then the "testing out" phase: are you doing things because you feel obligated? Did you start a volunteer project, join an association, or club only to find out it is not what you thought it was going to be? Does it require more time than you want to give, or has turned into something that no longer serves you?

I believe everyone has at least **one** thing you are doing that is taking time away from your life. Write it down, get a supportive friend (like Sandy) to share it with. Role play, and give it a timeline on when you will release it. Wait and see how relieved you feel! That will be the reward and the acknowledgment that you are making the right decision. End the year with cleaning off things, people, or situations that no longer serve you.

ACTION PLAN NO. 41

Power down for one week. Use this time to deepen your connections. Pick times as a family to unplug. Turn off televisions, computers, video games, tablets and other mobile devices. Have everyone sign a commitment contract to stay technology free for a week.

After you do this for one week, you may want to periodically unplug throughout the year. Turn off the technology for a week of digital detox!

[CHALLENGE 41] TURN OFF TECHNOLOGY

There are so many ways to stay connected these days. There are also many ways to express yourself through social media. You can literally lose hours scrolling through vast wastelands of Facebook pages and Instagram posts. How many times have you looked up a high school friend or someone from college you once knew to see how they are doing, and before you know it, it is midnight? Wasting away time that can be spent with the people you actually "see", like your children, husband, sister, brother or neighbors. Think of how actually spending time "communicating" would deepen your relationships on all levels.

Your family and friends want to know that you are excited to see them and in that moment, they need your eye contact. They need you to smile. They need you to listen and not say "one sec" and be put on hold.

Recently, I was out to dinner with my husband. Looking around at the people at the tables, I noticed that every single one of them had their faces down and phones or tablets in hand. Some were smiling and some looked mad. Still others looked as if they had zoned out and were not really aware of their surroundings. This is when I thought how powerful it would be to "turn off" the technology, even if it was for just one week. The impact it could have on real live relationships would be huge. Here are even more reasons for a digital detox:

Your brain will work better. You think you are multitasking, but in reality, your lack of focus on completion of a projects adds more stress and less efficiency.

Your communication with colleagues will improve. You may have experienced this at work... You are sitting in a meeting. Someone is explaining something you either already know or you don't need to know, so you wander over to your email or to your social media accounts. You read a few interesting messages and are just formulating a response when you suddenly realize that the talk of the meeting has shifted to something you very much need to know, but you missed an important point. Or worse, someone just asked you a question that did not register.

You will sleep better and wake up rested. If you sleep with your phone beside you and set on vibrate, you probably are not sleeping that soundly. People routinely tell me that they are woken up several times a night when their phone vibrates. Keeping your phone off at night, or better yet in another room, will help you get the rest you need.

You will get better at solving problems. Ever notice how many of your best ideas and most effective solutions to problems seem to come to you while you are doing something like taking a shower or going for a walk? There is a reason for that. Taking your direct attention away from constant interaction lets other parts of your brain go to work for you, with serious benefits. Allow your mind to have "zen moments".

[CHALLENGE 42] THE POWER OF ENCOURAGEMENT

There was a time in my life when I was feeling betrayed by those around me. In every corner of my life I felt abandoned; from family members, and from people who I had thought were my friends. During this dark time, I would stand next to strangers who were laughing… just so their joy could wash over me. When a cashier or clerk would say "have a nice day", I would wrap those words around me like a warm blanket, feeling comforted by their kindness.

Never before had I realized how powerful the energy of words could be, and it was eye-opening. You never know the impact that your words can have on strangers, friends, or family. When two people interact, they are both changed.

Whether our influence is helpful or hurtful, positive or negative, depends on whether we are giving the "gift" of encouragement. When you interact with someone, are you the encourager or discourager? Listen to your words, and see how it impacts your fellow human.

ACTION PLAN NO. 41

Spread encouraging words to everyone you interact with this week. A simple gesture, a "thank you" and a smile, or something larger.

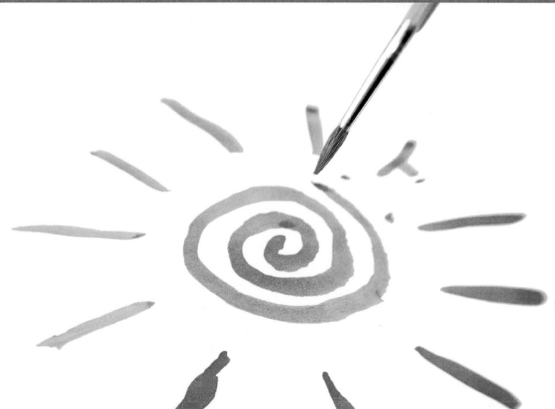

OCTOBER IN REVIEW

FOR OCTOBER
MY GOALS

FOR OCTOBER
MY GRATITUDE LIST

FOR OCTOBER
RELATIONSHIPS TO INVEST IN

FOR OCTOBER
WHAT'S GOING WELL

FOR OCTOBER
WHAT NEEDS TO CHANGE

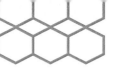

MY DOODLE SQUARE

NOVEMBER

LIFE COACHING / FITNESS / NUTRITION: GEARING UP FOR END-OF-YEAR SUCCESS

[CHALLENGE 43]
SAY 'NO' TO THE GOOD AND 'YES' TO THE GREAT

[CHALLENGE 44]
YOUR BRA AND OTHER IMPORTANT GEAR

[CHALLENGE 45]
MAKE TIME FOR 'YOU' WITH H.I.I.T. TRAINING

[CHALLENGE 46]
GO SUGAR-FREE

[CHALLENGE 46]
FRIDAY IS NOT A THREE-DAY AFFAIR

ACTION PLAN NO. 43

Pick and choose where you will go, who you will invite, and how your holiday will be. Write it down and make it a project plan or design a vision board around it. Keep it simple: both the plan and the execution!

Explain to people who pressure you that you are in the process of simplifying, and hopefully they will respect your decision. If not, stick to your guns. This is your life, and you do have a limited amount of holiday time… so what do you want yours to look like?

[CHALLENGE 43]
SAY 'NO' TO THE GOOD AND 'YES' TO THE GREAT

Our to-do lists are reaching a fever pitch as the holidays are in full blown swing. Shopping for your family, co-workers, teachers, friends, neighbors. Decorating, getting down the ornaments, wrapping the presents, putting up the Christmas lights (inside and out), putting up the tree.

Holiday parties, cocktail parties, cookie exchanges, ornament exchanges, club get-togethers, business holiday functions, entertaining. Not to mention getting together with family you might never EVER see except at the holidays… and unfortunately (or fortunately) there is a reason for that fact!

Traffic, fighting the extra influx of people into the transit system, malls, roadways, *all* trying to get to their destinations on time and their to-do lists "done".

Hey! I thought this was the time of joy, love, and peace… well where is it?!

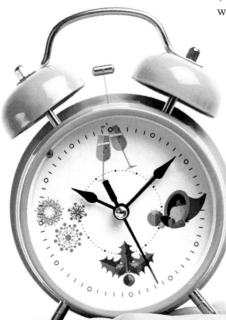

Stress is a part of life but during the holidays it peaks at an all-time high between the extra demands, extra alcohol, and extra calories! Emotions are frazzled and sleep is diminished. This is a recipe for stress and unhappiness! One more check in… if at the end of every holiday season, you are wiped out, unhappy, and even sick… then it is time for a change. It is time to make choices and say "no" to the good and "yes" to the great.

You can always start small by eliminating some things that suck the most life (joy) out of you and work backwards from there! This is a *big* challenge because of all the emotions wrapped around the holidays, but you deserve a life of happiness lived on your terms.

UNLESS YOU LIVE IN
PARADISE, IT'S ALL
ABOUT LAYERING AS
WINTER APPROACHES.

[CHALLENGE 44] YOUR BRA AND OTHER IMPORTANT GEAR

Let's talk about your bra. Yes, you read it right - your bra. We all know that eight out of ten women are wearing the wrong sized bra (thank you Oprah for telling us!). But did you know you may not be wearing the right sports bra?

The very first sports bra was literally two jock straps sewn together. Thirty-some years later, technology has come a long way! Scientists have figured out (finally!) that a sports bra needs to do more than stop up and down movement, it needs to take care of side to side movement as well. Most bras stop only up and down movement, which could be part of the reason more than half of women suffer breast pain during exercise. The right bra, however, can eliminate this pain for about 80 percent of women.

Most sports bras simply compress the breasts—not very comfortable and, in my opinion, not that attractive! A really good and supportive bra encapsulates each breast into its own cup (and of course, the cups have to be the right size!). Something else to think about: generally, a sports bra should be worn regularly for only about six months before it is replaced.

The weather is getting cooler, so don't forget to layer. Choose clothing layers of performance fabric that "wick" away the sweat. And an outer coat that is not only warm, but also waterproof. A warm hat and gloves are also a must. Keep a spare pair of gloves in your car so you won't ever forget.

ACTION PLAN NO. 44

Gear yourself up for success from the skin out. Unsupported, the average A cup breast travels about an inch and a half in each direction, and a D cup bounces two to three inches. A good sports bra can cut that movement in half, which is key to sparing the support structures in your breast. For the very best fit, don't rely on your everyday bra size. Get yourself fitted for a new sports bra and feel the difference! Can't get to a fitting? Here's the basics to do it yourself.

THREE EASY STEPS TO FIND YOUR PERFECT FIT

STEP 1 RIB MEASUREMENT Measure around your rib cage at the bottom band, just under the breast. The tape measure should feel quite snug. Round the measurement down to the closest inch.

STEP 2 BUST MEASUREMENT While wearing your everyday bra, that doesn't minimize or include padding, measure the bust over the fullest point of the breast. For larger-breasted women, the fullest point may not be at center, and is often lower. As breast tissue can fluctuate as much as 20%, round up to the closest inch.

STEP 3 CUP SIZE Subtract your rib measurement (step 1) from your bust measurement (step 2). Use the resulting number [the difference between Step 1 and Step 2] to determine your cup size as follows:

Difference	1″	2″	3″	4″	5″	6″
Cup size	A	B	C	D	DD/E	DDD/F

FITTING TIPS AND TRICKS

✓ Sports bras should fit slightly tighter than a regular bra, but not so tight that you can't comfortably take a deep breath with the bra fastened on the middle hook.

✓ There should be no chafing around the armholes, shoulder straps or seams. If the sports bra has hooks or snaps, make sure those don't chafe, either.

✓ The straps shouldn't dig into your shoulders.

✓ Test the bra's support by jumping or running in place. You'll be able to feel whether it's sufficiently supportive or not.

Divide and conquer... encapsulate each breast for the most comfortable support!

STRETCH

[CHALLENGE 45]
TIME FOR YOU WITH H.I.I.T. TRAINING

H.I.I.T., A.K.A. HIGH INTENSITY INTERVAL TRAINING, IS AN EXERCISE STRATEGY ALTERNATING SHORT PERIODS OF INTENSE ANAEROBIC EXERCISE WITH LESS-INTENSE RECOVERY PERIODS.

Coming into the holiday season and extra responsibilities, the first thing to usually go is any sort of "me" time! This includes work out time. Just when you need it the most with all the extra demands and stress! This is a trick I use for when I get really busy. Adding H.I.I.T. to your workout arsenal is wonderful for a lot of reasons.

WHY INTERVAL TRAINING?!

SUPER EFFICIENT 15 to 20 minutes is all you need! This is great for the time crunched holidays. You can squeeze in a workout between your busy day or even at lunch!

BURN MORE FAT Studies show you not only burn more calories but also more fat! Bonus: you push your body into overdrive, burning more calories and fat for the next 24 hours afterwards!

HEALTHIER HEART Most people aren't used to pushing themselves into their anaerobic zone (that lovely feeling when you push yourself so hard you feel like your heart is going to jump out of your chest). But in this case, it definitely produces results! Heart health improves dramatically after just a few short months of H.I.I.T. workouts.

NO EQUIPMENT NEEDED Running and/or jumping only requires you and your body so it is convenient and inexpensive!

LOSE WEIGHT, NOT MUSCLE As you know, muscle is your calorie burning engine, so you want to hold onto as much as possible! This short intense training encourages energy to be used from fat stores.

INCREASE METABOLIC RATE H.I.I.T. training increases production of HGH (human growth hormone) by 450% during the 24 hours after your workout. This is great news since HGH not only speeds up your metabolism, but also slows down the aging process, making you younger both inside and out!

YOURSELF WITH INTERVALS

MOJO NO. 1 H.I.I.T. WORKOUT

DO EACH EXERCISE FOR 45 SECONDS.
REST FOR 10 SECONDS BETWEEN EACH. @ 10X

[**JUMPING JACKS**] (modification: motions only without jump)

[**PUSHUPS**] (modification: knees down)

[**SQUATS**]

[**DIPS**]

[**LUNGES**]

[**HIGH KNEES**] walk like you are marching with knees as high as they will go

[**WALL SIT**]

MOJO NO. 2 H.I.I.T. WORKOUT

DO EACH EXERCISE FOR 60 SECONDS.
REST FOR 10 SECONDS BETWEEN EACH. @ 10X

[**CENTER PLANK**]

[**JUMPING JACKS**] (modification: motions only without jump)

[**SIDE PLANK: RIGHT SIDE**]

[**SQUAT HOPS**]

[**SIDE PLANK: LEFT SIDE**]

[**SQUAT HOPS**]

[**PUSHUPS**]

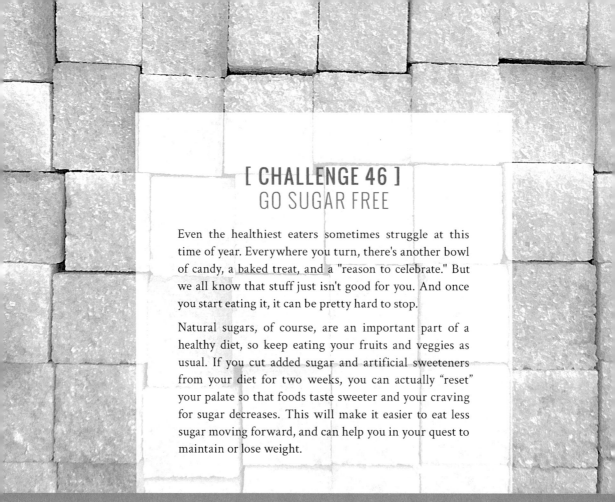

[CHALLENGE 46]
GO SUGAR FREE

Even the healthiest eaters sometimes struggle at this time of year. Everywhere you turn, there's another bowl of candy, a baked treat, and a "reason to celebrate." But we all know that stuff just isn't good for you. And once you start eating it, it can be pretty hard to stop.

Natural sugars, of course, are an important part of a healthy diet, so keep eating your fruits and veggies as usual. If you cut added sugar and artificial sweeteners from your diet for two weeks, you can actually "reset" your palate so that foods taste sweeter and your craving for sugar decreases. This will make it easier to eat less sugar moving forward, and can help you in your quest to maintain or lose weight.

ACTION PLAN NO. 46

This week, give yourself a jump start on the holidays by eliminating the refined sugar from your diet. No soda, no cookies, no ice cream... and don't even think about that candy. But you weren't eating that stuff anyway, right?! One week: no refined sugar. You **can** do it, and your body will love you for it.

[CHALLENGE 47] FRIDAY IS NOT A THREE-DAY AFFAIR

It is Friday. The office is going for Mexican food. All week long, you have avoided the treats in the break room. Ignored the ice cream your husband or roommate brought home. You have been on your game! And now it is Friday and the office is celebrating the ending of a huge project that you have been responsible for. You have to go right?!?

In addition, you forgot your Grab 'N Go's and thought it was no big deal; after all it is Friday! Two margaritas and a basket of chips later, you decide you might as well order the combo plate and start over on Monday! So the weekend turns into a free-for-all, with you eating and drinking your way through Saturday and Sunday. You wake up on Monday feeling totally defeated, puffy, and depressed. Not the best way to start your week!

Wow! There are so many things going on with this story but we are going to focus on one thing... it was *only Friday*! It was only one meal! "Stinking thinking" got you into a spiraling vortex of indulgence that you could not stop! No need to continue with one slip-up through the weekend. In Mama Bootcamp land, we start over once the meal is done. That means getting up Saturday morning and getting to your Bootcamp! Hopefully you pounded some water before bedtime to start the flushing process. Then the weekend can be all about "clean eating" and having fun with movement (a.k.a. exercising)!

ACTION PLAN NO. 47

Realize when you might be at risk. Remember you have tools to assist you.

TOOLS TO STAY ON TRACK

✓ Pre-plan and pre-pack your Grab 'N Go's to keep your blood sugar stable so you do not feel like eating the wall paper (or the bag of chips in the pantry) when you come through the door.

✓ On your way to a "risky" event (that has all of your favorite foods), eat an apple and drink a large bottle of water. The soluble fiber in the apple will expand to help fill you up! And "double bam", you will not be dehydrated! People mistake hunger for thirst all the time!

✓ Eat every two to four hours. You do not want to skip lunch because you are going out to your favorite restaurant! You do not want to eat like a Sumo wrestler right?! So eat your clean and healthy lunch and move on.

✓ If you have had a hard day or emotional day right before the weekend, seek out friends who support you instead of diving into a box of donuts. Find the support you need in friends or family. Plan events that bring you joy and/or comfort. I have heard from 90% of my Mamas, "I am an emotional eater." Well, welcome to the club! We celebrate, mourn, love, cry, laugh all round food! Most events, whether it is a funeral or a birthday, involve food! In addition, if you know chocolate is your addiction, then please do not have it on the house. Keep your home your haven and your oasis of peacefulness. No wrestling with "should I eat that or not" at 10 p.m. at night!

✓ Try your best to do away with "perfection performance"! Cut yourself some slack! I hate to be the one to tell you, but you are not perfect. If you were, you would not be here. You are a person who is going to fall down once a while. So pick yourself back up, dust yourself off, and keep moving.

✓ You need to treat yourself like you would a dear friend. Your negative self-talk can walk you right into a weekend of binge eating. Do not beat yourself up for not being "perfect". Why didn't I just stay on track? What is wrong with me? Why can't I just say no? I will always be fat! And on and on and on... so self- destructive. Remember, it was just one meal.

✓ You know it has been a tough week and you are vulnerable. Plan an active weekend that will help you decompress. An exercise group (power in numbers), a fun run, hike, bowling, a day at the lake or river, all will help you to burn off the stress and anxiety of a long week.

NOVEMBER IN REVIEW

FOR NOVEMBER
MY GOALS

FOR NOVEMBER
MY GRATITUDE LIST

FOR NOVEMBER
RELATIONSHIPS TO INVEST IN

FOR NOVEMBER
WHAT'S GOING WELL

FOR NOVEMBER
WHAT NEEDS TO CHANGE

NOVEMBER NOTES

MY DOODLE SQUARE

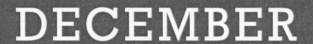

DECEMBER

LIFE COACHING: UNWRAPPING THE HOLIDAYS

[CHALLENGE 48] "WHAT'S YOUR EXCUSE?"

We all have them...the voices in our heads that come up with amazing reasons not to work out, to procrastinate on a project, or to avoid someone we promised to spend time with. These voices are excuses, and we really all do have them and heed them more than we should.

How are your excuses preventing you from living your best life? How do your excuses steal you Mojo?

If you are having a hard time getting motivated, or staying motivated, take a look at why. What are *your* excuses and why are you sabotaging yourself? When you have a wedding or a reunion, have you noticed how determined you are? Nothing will get in your way of fitting into that special dress. Nothing stands in the way of you finding your "mojo".

ACTION PLAN NO. 48

Listen to the voices that make up your excuses and hear what they are saying. Write them all down. Then come up with a strategy to defeat them. Use rewards, the buddy system (work out partner or group), an accountability partner (can be your BFF even in another city) who you text when you've completed your workout, set a goal like your first 5K or triathlon (that will get you moving), or even a simple mantra to break through your excuses.

Mantras need to be simple and in first person – claiming it to be so. These are examples of possible mantras for you:

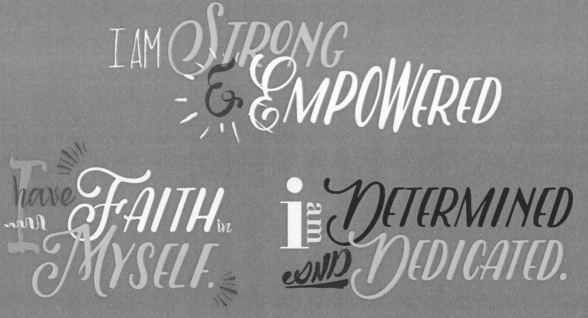

I AM STRONG & EMPOWERED

I have FAITH in MYSELF.

i am DETERMINED and DEDICATED.

Remember this: If something is truly important to you, you will find a way to make it happen. If it isn't truly important, you can always find an excuse.

[CHALLENGE 49]
WHAT YOU THINK OF ME IS NONE OF MY BUSINESS

It's 2007... I am in a business that I built from the ground up. It had been years in the making, and a dream come true for me... until the doors were opened.

From the outside, my business looked like Shangri-La... an oasis. But internally, it was full of lies; dysfunction and back stabbing. I was working with a business partner who could rationalize the most unethical behavior. My talent and abilities were being undermined and self-doubt crept in. The negativity was literally eating a hole in me, and I was constantly getting sick! I did not understand how people could be so cruel to one another and justify it.

I went to my husband and told him I was leaving the business and wasn't sure what I wanted to do. I was not sure if I wanted to stay in the health and fitness industry. I knew if I stayed where I was at, I would surely die. The job was sucking the life out of me. He totally supported my decision to leave.

When I left, malicious gossip began to float around, and I started hearing about it. The drama was still continuing to affect me even after leaving. I was having a hard time healing from the loss of my dream, until one day someone said to me:

"Their opinion of you, is none of your business. Keep walking your walk and continue to be true to yourself."

When I heard this, a sense of relief washed over me. It was like someone applied ointment to an open wound. Those words helped me let go, so I could heal. I was relieved of the responsibility of responding

ACTION PLAN NO. 49

Are you being sucked in to someone else's gossip and rumors? Think about the times during the day where you are going over and over what someone said to you OR what you heard someone say about you.

Ask yourself "why did she say that?" Make a point to say to yourself, what she/he thinks of me is none of my business. And remind yourself that you must be pretty important for someone to spend their time talking about you. Don't waste your energy on things that have no importance in your life. Everyone is going to have an opinion... some different than yours. The biggest and most important point is: are you being true to yourself?

to all of the negative talk I was hearing. I allowed myself to truly let it go! There was a huge sense of closure... it truly was *none of my business.*

I use this wonderful advice to this day, and have even taken it a step further. If they are talking about you, then you must be pretty important! Honestly, you are never going to have everyone agree with you, or even like you. Each person has their own opinion of how you are living, but if you are true to yourself and doing what you know is right for you and your life, you will be happy and at peace... both equally important!

[CHALLENGE 50]
YOU ARE STRONGER THAN YOU KNOW

I was out for a bike ride with a few women, all of us just starting back on our bikes after a long cold winter. We had planned our first long hilly ride for the season. One incredibly strong, fit woman, Sue, was doubting herself (probably like we all were) and said "I don't know if I can do the hills so I will just take it slow and if I need to, I will turn around and just go back." We assured her we were all feeling the same way and we would stick together! And sure enough, at the peak of the hill, Sue said "I had no idea I could do that and I almost did not come! Not only did I do it, but I feel great!"

Where do you doubt yourself and give up *before* you even try? I bet there are a few places or situations and things you have missed out on because you were in doubt.

ACTION PLAN NO. 50

Squeeze you hand into a fist: as tight as you can!... then wait a few seconds and squeeze even tighter. I bet you did squeeze a little tighter. You can almost always do just a tiny bit more than you are giving yourself credit for!

The next time any self-doubt creeps in, squeeze your hand into a fist and tell yourself that you are stronger than you know.

[CHALLENGE 51] BRAIN OVERLOAD: TAKE TIME TO BREATHE

How many times have you been running around your house, late for work, looking for your keys? Heck, you had driven home last night….they *have* to be here somewhere!!! Frantically, the clock is ticking by and you are running later and later. Only to find them right where you put them! This, my friends, is called "brain overload". The culmination of too many responsibilities, projects, calendars, meetings, time constraints, stress, appointments, and pressure! You cannot possible handle *one* more thing!

I had an extreme case of brain overload when my three children were little. Life was stressful. I was pretty much a single parent. The children's dad was working in California while I lived in Oregon. I was managing the kids, the home, working part time at the local hospital teaching chair aerobics to patients, plus working at a local health club. At the same time, I was struggling to come to terms with my relationship with my mother. To say I was a little stressed is an understatement. I was squeezing in a grocery shopping trip between duties. I had finished loading all the groceries in the back of the van without closing the back door of the van. I drove away from the store and down the street. As I left, a trail of toilet paper, apples, cereal, milk, etc. falling out of my van behind me.

Definitely brain overload! If I had known then what I know now, I would have taken a few minutes to decompress and catch my breath.

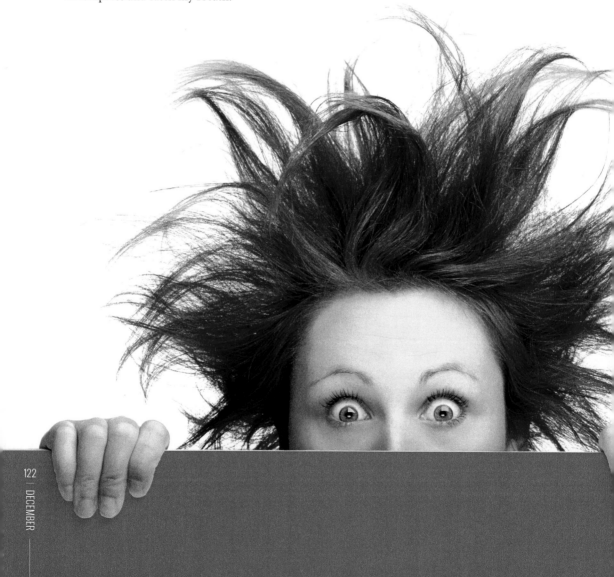

I am sure you have similar situations that have happened in the past or are happening now. I suggest taking it one step further and add a daily meditation. I can hear you now... "But I barely have time to breathe *now*! And you want me to add something onto my calendar?"

With meditation, the physiology of your body undergoes a change and every cell in the body is filled with more prana (energy). This results in joy, peace, enthusiasm as the level of prana in the body increases. Additionally, Meditation brings the brainwave pattern into an Alpha state that promotes healing. The mind becomes fresh, energized and recharged.

MEDITATION ROCKS!

MORE PHYSICAL BENEFITS OF MEDITATION

Lowers high blood pressure

Decreases any tension-related pain, such as tension headaches, ulcers, insomnia

Increases serotonin production that improves mood and behavior

Improves the immune system

Increases the energy level, as you gain an inner source of energy

AND MORE MENTAL BENEFITS OF MEDITATION

Anxiety decreases

Emotional stability improves

Creativity increases

Happiness increases

Gain clarity and peace of mind

Problems become smaller

So many benefits for a minimal time investment! This will help you handle the challenges of life in a graceful, thoughtful way before you lose your keys or your groceries!

ACTION PLAN NO. 51

Set up a time daily to meditate that will not be forgotten or ignored. The first thing in the morning is great. You want to establish this as new daily habit, so it needs to be a priority. Here is a simple meditation for beginners.

1. **Sit or lie comfortably. Pick the same place daily so your body and brain knows when it goes to this place, you are preparing to meditate.**

2. **Close your eyes.**

3. **Make no effort to control the breath; simply breathe naturally.**

4. **Focus your attention on the breath and on how the body moves with each inhalation and exhalation. Notice the movement of your body as you breathe. Observe your chest, shoulders, rib cage and belly. Make no effort to control your breath; simply focus your attention. If your mind wanders, simply return your focus back to your breath. Maintain this meditation practice for 2–3 minutes to start, and then try it for longer periods.**

Super simple right? And the benefits are huge! Make a plan. Put it on your calendar and make it a priority! Love this weekly challenge for it is such a simple concept with huge returns for your time.

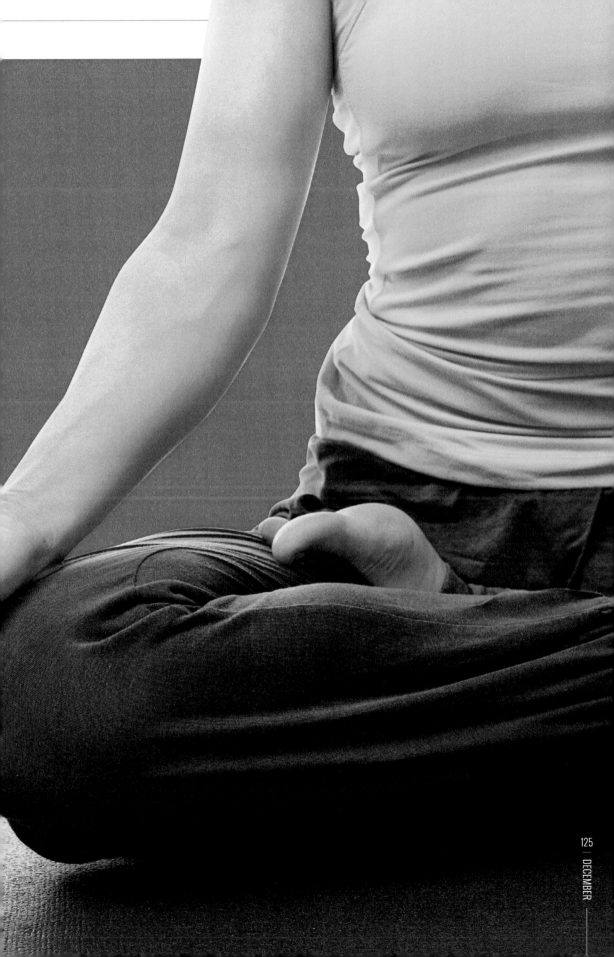

[CHALLENGE 52] WHAT ARE YOU THANKFUL FOR?

What you focus on grows… so what are you focusing on? Past hurts or pains? Or positive experiences? People who have been blessings in your life? What you think about comes about, so start creating by having an attitude of gratitude! Be thankful for things large and small: a smile from a stranger, your job. And why would God give you anything more if you are not thankful for what you have.

In 1999, when I first left my abusive husband, I was very anxious about raising three very small children all under six years old. Their father was arrested for hitting me and breaking down the front door. With no child support and no job, I applied for welfare. I had zero dollars to my name. Praying for help, I decided to get my children out of the house for a walk as the sun had just come out. Walking down the street, I started to see sparkles on the ground. As I got closer, I realized someone had thrown *lots* of change all over the road!

MY DOODLE SQUARE

We all started happily picking up all the pennies! I told my children they were "pennies from heaven" and that was God's way of telling us everything was going to be alright.

Blessings happen all the time… are you thankful or unaware? If you are not thankful, why would God give you any more? Create an energy of thankfulness and watch what happens. Abundance and prosperity is created in those moments!

ACTION PLAN NO. 52

Start a gratitude journal and write three things you are thankful for every day! Start with the small things: your favorite pillow, your best friend, a favorite song. Go back and read your journal after several days and you will realize the abundance you have in your life.

DECEMBER IN REVIEW

FOR DECEMBER
MY GOALS

FOR DECEMBER
MY GRATITUDE LIST

FOR DECEMBER
RELATIONSHIPS TO INVEST IN

FOR DECEMBER
WHAT'S GOING WELL

FOR DECEMBER
WHAT NEEDS TO CHANGE